MW01014501

THE PA BIBLE

*A PANCE Workbook Written
by the Physician Assistants
Who Wished They'd Had It*

Christine Nelson,

Tiffany Lee,

&

Meredith Allen

The PA Bible: A PANCE Workbook Written by the Physician Assistants Who Wished They'd Had It

Copyright ©2023 CHRISTINE NELSON. All rights reserved.

No part of this book may be reproduced in any form or by any mechanical means, including information storage and retrieval systems without permission in writing from the publisher/author, except by a reviewer who may quote passages in a review. All images, logos, quotes, and trademarks included in this book are subject to use according to trademark and copyright laws of the United States of America.

NELSON, CHRISTINE, Author
THE PA BIBLE
CHRISTINE NELSON

In Association with:
ELITE ONLINE PUBLISHING
63 East 11400 South #230
Sandy, UT 84070
EliteOnlinePublishing.com

ISBN: 978-1-956642-41-4 (Paperback)
MED058210
MED086000

QUANTITY PURCHASES: Schools, companies, professional groups, clubs,
and other organizations may qualify for special terms when ordering quantities of this title. For information, email
info@ eliteonlinepublishing.com.

All rights reserved by CHRISTINE NELSON and ELITE ONLINE PUBLISHING
This book is printed in the United States of America.

Why We Created This Workbook

Our hope is that PA students can have most everything needed to study for the PANCE in one place, this workbook. While studying for the PANCE ourselves we spent hundreds of dollars on different books and online systems and felt overwhelmed by the options and at times too much information. We wanted to create a workbook that was directly tailored to the PANCE blueprint, user-friendly, and concise enough as to not be overwhelming. This workbook is specifically designed to categorize necessary information while allowing the student to participate in the process by filling in the information, which has been proven to help with recall and retention.

How to Use This Workbook

- We recognize some of the topics fit into multiple subjects, but we kept it simple by only putting each topic in one place in the workbook. You can find each topic in the appendix if it isn't where you instinctively think it would be.

- Some topics may not have enough room to put everything in that you learn. We recommend putting in the information that is harder to remember, and not writing what you already know. This will help to ensure that your individual workbook doesn't become overcrowded or busy.

- There are "empty" boxes within the workbook that are intended for the reader to draw or fill in that information, again this helps with recollection and learning.

- There is a section at the end of each chapter to put the most commonly used medications within each subject.

- There are also lined pages at the end of each subject so that you can add any subjects or information that you feel are important but that aren't specifically on the PANCE blueprint.

Table of Contents

Cardiology

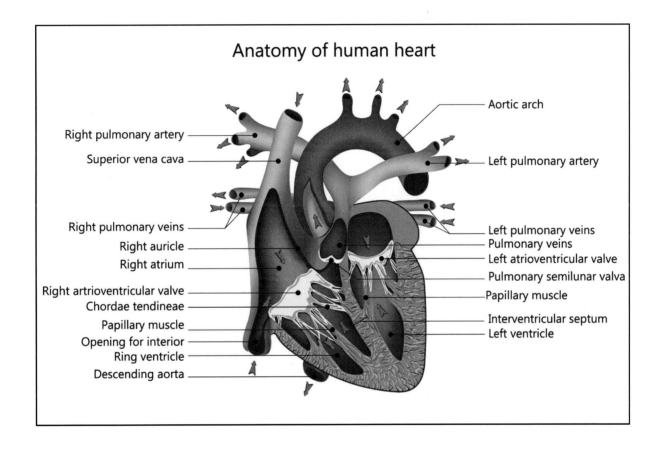

Anatomy of human heart

Right pulmonary artery

Superior vena cava

Right pulmonary veins

Right auricle

Right atrium

Right artrioventricular valve

Chordae tendineae

Papillary muscle

Opening for interior

Ring ventricle

Descending aorta

Aortic arch

Left pulmonary artery

Left pulmonary veins

Pulmonary veins

Left atrioventricular valve

Pulmonary semilunar valva

Papillary muscle

Interventricular septum

Left ventricle

Inflammatory Cardiac Disorders

Pericarditis: Most common viral (coxsackie), autoimmune

Sx:

PE: Pericardial friction rub, squeaking sound on auscultation

Dx: Serum troponin, echocardiogram, Chest X-ray, and EKG showing diffuse ST elevation

_____

_____

_____

Tx:

PERICARDITIS

a healthy pericardium   pericarditis

Dressler's Syndrome: Immune response to damaged heart muscle (type of pericarditis)

Sx:

PE:

Dx: CBC shows increased WBC, CRP, & ESR

_____

_____

_____

Tx:

Pericardial Effusion: Fluid in pericardial space - can lead to cardiac tamponade

Sx:

PE: Tachycardia, tachypnea, hypotension, elevated jugular venous pressure

Dx:

_____

_____

_____

Tx:

QRS wave electric alternation
QRS wave amplitude and shape alternately

Cardiac Tamponade: Compression of all heart chambers resulting in narrow pulse pressure, pulsus paradoxus

Sx:

PE: BECKS TRIAD =

Dx: Transthoracic echocardiogram, Chest X-ray, CBC, cardiac enzymes

_____   Tx:

_____

_____

Myocarditis: Cardiac muscle inflammation - can lead to CHF
Causes: Cocaine use, post viral illness in young patients = parvovirus/coxsackie

Sx:

PE:

Dx: Elevated cardiac enzymes

_____   Tx:

_____

_____

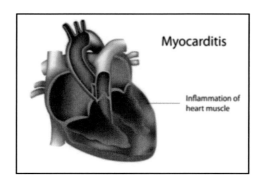

Endocarditis: Fever + new murmur
IV drug use = S. aureus (affects tricuspid)
GI cancer = Strep bovis or gallolyticus

Sx: Fever, anorexia, Roth Spots, Osler Nodes, murmur, Janeway Lesions, anemia, splinter
  hemorrhages

PE:

Dx: CBC, echocardiogram, EKG, blood cultures

_____   Tx:

_____

_____

<u>Dukes Criteria</u>

Major Criteria:

Minor Criteria:

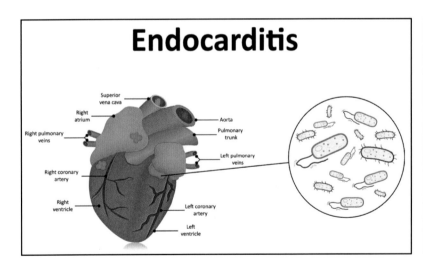

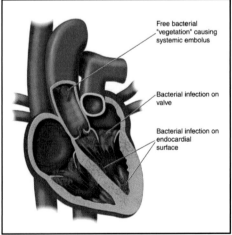

Valvular Disorders

Aortic Stenosis:

Causes: Congenital bicuspid, rheumatic fever, age, calcifications

Sx:

Murmur:

Dx: Transthoracic echocardiogram, EKG, Chest X-ray

_____   **Tx:**

_____

_____

Aortic Regurgitation:

Causes: Marfan's Syndrome, rheumatic fever, aortic dilation

Sx: Depends on severity and cause

Murmur:

Dx:

_____   **Tx:**

_____

_____

Mitral Stenosis:
Causes: Rheumatic fever

Sx:

Murmur:

Dx: Transthoracic echocardiogram, EKG, Chest X-ray

_____

_____

_____

Tx:

Mitral Regurgitation (Acute and Chronic):
Acute = sudden volume overload, acute pulmonary edema
Causes: mitral valve prolapse, ischemia

Sx: Dyspnea with exertion, lower extremity edema, fatigue

Murmur:

Dx:

_____

_____

_____

Tx:

Mitral Valve Prolapse:
Risk Factors: Connective tissue disorders

Sx:

Murmur:

Dx: Transthoracic echocardiogram & transesophageal echocardiogram

_____

_____

_____

Tx:

Pulmonary Stenosis: **Can lead to right heart failure**

Sx:

Murmur:

Dx: Echocardiogram

_____   **Tx:**

_____

_____

Pulmonary Regurgitation:

Sx:

Murmur:

Dx: Echocardiogram

_____   **Tx:**

_____

_____

Tricuspid Stenosis:

Causes: Rheumatic fever, IV drug use

Sx:

Murmur:

Dx: Echocardiogram

_____   **Tx:**

_____

_____

Tricuspid Regurgitation: **Can be asymptomatic**

Cause: IV drug use

Sx:

Murmur:

Dx: Echocardiogram

_____   **Tx:**

_____

_____

Rheumatic Fever: **Strep**

Sx: Jones Criteria

PE:

Dx:

_____   **Tx:**

_____

_____

Jones Criteria	
Major Criteria	Minor Criteria

Systolic Murmurs

Diastolic Murmurs

Innocent Murmur:

Sx:

PE:

Dx: Echocardiogram with color doppler

_____

_____

_____

Stills Murmurs (Type of Innocent Murmur):

Sx: Asymptomatic

PE:

Dx:

_____

_____

_____

Cervical Venous Hum (Type of Innocent Murmur):

Sx: Asymptomatic

PE:

Dx: Echocardiogram

_____

_____

_____

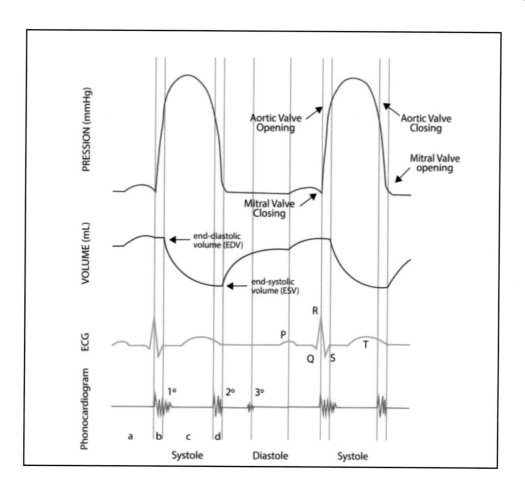

Murmur Vocabulary

Carvallo's sign = murmurs are louder with inhalation

Stenosis = not able to fully open

S1 = closure of Mitral & Tricuspid valves

S2 = closure of Atrial & Pulmonic valves

S3 = ventricular overload (rapid filling)

S4 = decreased LV wall compliance (atrial contraction)

Splitting = asynchrony between AV or semilunar valves

Click = abrupt halting of valve - leaflet folding into the atrium & suddenly stopped by chordae tendinea

Thrill = palpable murmur - feels like a vibration

Heave = abnormally large beating of the heart - sign of LVH

Diaphragm = increased pitched sounds (normal heart sounds & systolic murmurs)

Bell = decreased pitched sounds (S3, S4, diastolic murmurs, bruits)

Acute Coronary Syndrome

Stable Angina:

Risk Factors: Smoking, hypertension, diabetes, obesity

Sx: Pain with exertion that resolves with rest

PE:

Dx: Exercise stress test, EKG, HbA1c, normal troponin, & CK-MB

_____   **Tx:**

_____

_____

Unstable Angina:

Risk Factors: Smoking, hypertension, diabetes, obesity, hyperlipidemia

Sx: Pain at rest, may not be relieved with nitroglycerin

PE:

Dx: Normal cardiac enzymes, EKG, Chest X-ray, coronary angiography

_____   **Tx:**

_____

_____

Prinzmetal Angina: Coronary spasms

Risk Factors: Smoking, young

Sx: Mostly in the morning time

PE:

Dx: EKG with ST elevations, coronary angiography

_____   **Tx:**

_____

_____

NSTEMI:

Sx:

PE:

Dx: Elevated troponin and CK–MB, EKG = ST depression

_____   **Tx:**

_____

_____

STEMI:

Sx:

PE:

Dx: EKG = ST elevation

_____   **Tx:**

_____

_____

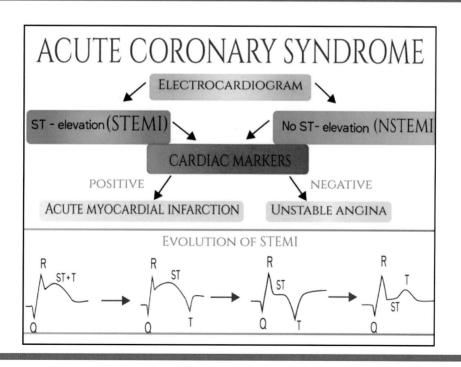

Acute Myocardial Infarction

Anterior MI

Tx:

Inferior & Right Ventricle MI

Tx:

Do not use nitroglycerin, morphine, or Viagra

Lateral MI

Tx:

Posterior MI

Tx:

Beck's Triad = decreased BP, clear lungs, JVD

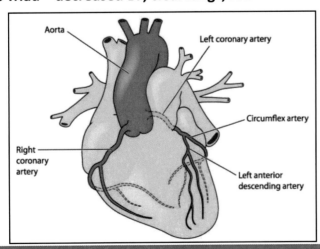

Post MI Care

Aspirin 81 mg QD (clopidogrel if allergy)

ACEI or ARB - to improve left ventricular ejection fraction

BB - decreased mortality by decreased O2 demand
 Prolong diastole to improve coronary flow
 Decreased chance for V-fib
 Avoid with: Bronchospasm, hypotensive & unstable, Heart block > 1ˢᵗ degree, heart failure

Fiber

Statins - stabilize plaques
 LDL < 70

Combined aspirin/clopidogrel - use 6-12 months in stented pts

Lifestyle changes = quit tobacco, increase dietary fiber, decrease saturated fat, increase weight loss

Cardiac Rehab = medically monitored cardiovascular exercise
 Stimulated angiogenesis
 Decreased post-MI depression

Dysrhythmias & Conduction Disorders

1st Degree Heart Block: **Delay @ AV node**

Dx: EKG = PR interval > 0.2

_____

_____

Tx:

First Degree AV Block

2nd Degree Heart Block: **Mobitz I, Wenckebach**

Dx: EKG = PR interval longer each cycle then drops

_____

_____

Tx:

Second degree AV block (Mobitz I)

2nd Degree Heart Block: **Mobitz II - not benign - conduction system disease below Bundle of HIS**

Dx: EKG = normal or long PR with dropped QRS

_____

_____

Tx:

Second degree AV block (Mobitz II)

3rd Degree Heart Block: **Complete heart block - severe bradycardia due to absence of AV node conduction**

Dx: EKG = independent atrial and ventricular rhythms
with widened QRS complex

Cannon A wave =

_____

_____

Tx:

Third degree AV block

BUNDLE BRANCH BLOCK: Often asymptomatic - ventricular depolarization takes longer
Right Bundle Branch Block: Rule out pulmonary embolism

Bunny ears in pre-cordial leads
Slurred S waves in lateral leads

Dx:

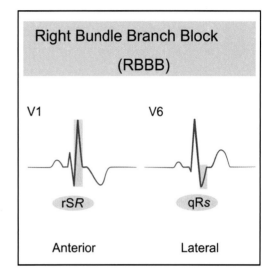

Tx:

Left Bundle Branch Block: Rule out myocardial infarction

Absence of Q wave in lead 1, V5, & V6
Monomorphic R wave displaced opposite QRS complex

Dx:

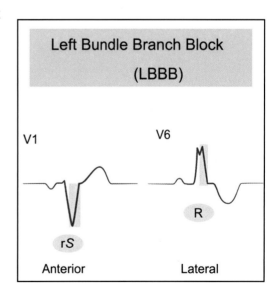

Tx:

Sick Sinus Syndrome: **Sinoatrial node dysfunction**

Sx:

PE:

Dx: EKG = bradycardia, sinus pause, sinus arrest

Tx:

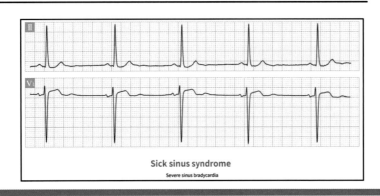

Sick sinus syndrome
Severe sinus bradycardia

Premature Beats

Tx:

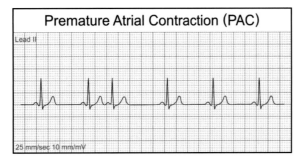

Tx:

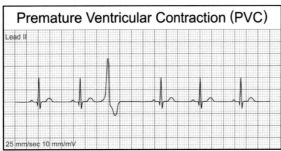

Tx:

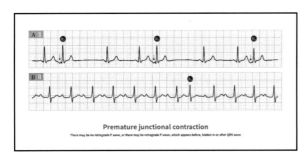

Premature junctional contraction
There may be no retrograde P wave, or there may be retrograde P wave, which appears before, hidden in or after QRS wave

Sinus Arrythmia:

Sx: Usually asymptomatic

PE:

Dx: EKG

_____   **Tx:**

_____

_____

Atrial Fibrillation: Irregularly irregular

Sx: Palpitations, hypotension, irregular pulse rate

PE:

Dx:

_____   **Tx:**

_____

_____

Atrial Flutter:

Sx:

PE:

Dx: EKG sawtooth pattern

_____

_____

_____

Tx:

Supraventricular Tachycardia:

Sx: Palpitations, abrupt onset & termination

PE:

Dx:

_____

_____

_____

Tx:

Supraventricular Tachycardia (SVT)
Lead II

25 mm/sec 10 mm/mV

Wolf Parkinson White: **Bundle of Kent**

Sx:

PE:

Dx: EKG = delta waves

_____

_____

_____

Draw the rhythm

Tx:

Long QT:

Sx:

PE:

Dx: EKG = long QT interval

_____

_____

_____

Draw the rhythm

Tx:

Ventricular Tachycardia:

Most common cause:

Sx:

PE:

Dx: 3 or more PVCs, HR > 120

Ventricular Tachycardia

Tx:

_____

_____

_____

Torsades de Pointes:

Most common cause: Hypomagnesaemia

Sx:

PE:

Dx: EKG = twisting around base

Tx:

_____

_____

_____

Ventricular Fibrillation: **Quivering of ventricles**

Sx:

PE:

Dx: EKG

Tx:

_____

_____

_____

Ventricular Fibrillation

Vascular Disorders

Chronic Peripheral Arterial Disease:

Sx: Claudication, weak pedal pulses, leg hair stops growing, lower leg ulcers

PE:

Dx: US, arteriography, ankle brachial index < 0.90

_____   Tx:

_____

_____

Acute Peripheral Arterial Disease: **Limb occlusion**

Sx: 6 Ps (pain, pallor, poikilothermia, pulselessness, paresthesia, and paralysis)

PE:

Dx:

_____   Tx:

_____

_____

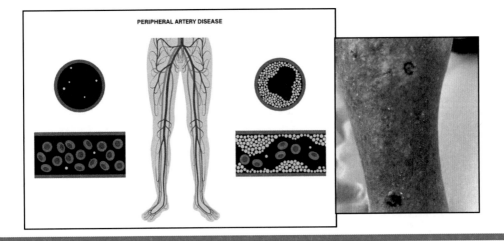

Abdominal Aortic Aneurysm:

Risk Factors: Age, smoking

Sx:

PE: Pulsatile mass

Dx:

_____   Tx:

_____

_____

Thoracic Aortic Aneurysm:

Sx: Dyspnea, dysphagia, cough, hoarseness

PE:

Dx: Angiography

_____   Tx:

_____

_____

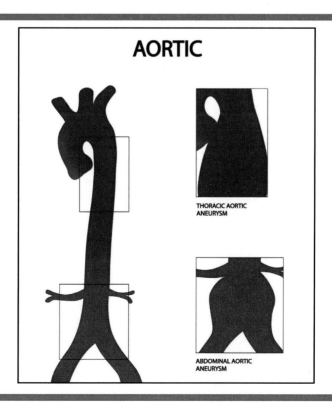

Aortic Dissection:

Sx: Tear of intima, ripping chest pain, decreased asymmetric pulses

Type A = proximal

Type B = distal

PE:

Dx: CT, MRA, transesophageal echocardiogram, Chest X-ray with widening of mediastinum

Tx:

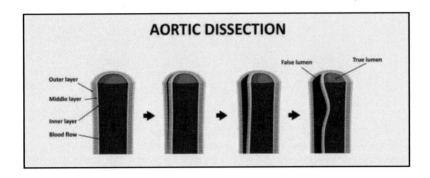

Arteriovenous Malformation (AVM): **Brain & peripheral**

Sx:

PE:

Dx: Vascular imaging (angiography)

Tx:

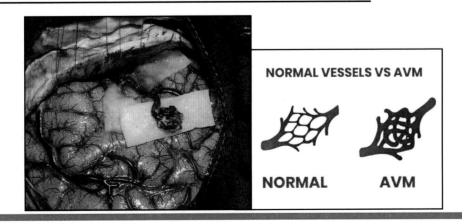

Giant Cell (Temporal) Arteritis: Associated with polymyalgia rheumatica

Sx: Headache, jaw claudication, tender, vision loss

PE:

Dx: ESR > 100, temporal artery biopsy

_____   Tx:

_____

_____

Deep Vein Thrombosis (DVT):

Sx: Pain, erythema

PE: Positive Homan's sign

Dx:

| **Virchow's Triad** |
| **Stasis, hypercoagulable, trauma** |

_____   Tx:

_____

_____

Superficial Vein Thrombophlebitis (Phlebitis): Inflammation leading to clot

Sx:

PE: Palpable cord

Dx: Venous US

_____   Tx:

_____

_____

Acute Mesenteric Ischemia:

Sx: Sudden abdominal pain

PE:

Dx: CTA, MRA, or CT without contrast

_____ **Tx:**

_____

_____

Chronic Mesenteric Ischemia:

Sx: Postprandial pain

PE:

Dx: CTA, MRA, or duplex US

_____ **Tx:**

_____

_____

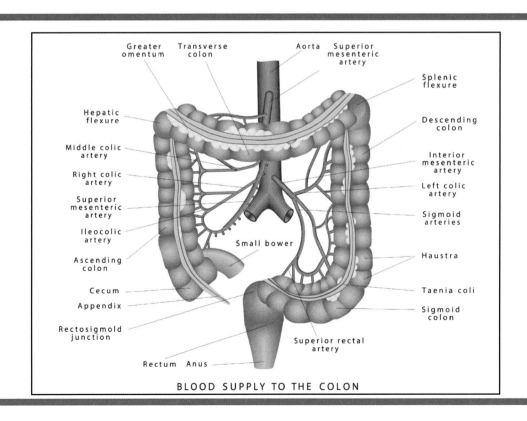

BLOOD SUPPLY TO THE COLON

Buerger's Disease (Thromboangiitis Obliterans): Inflammatory vasculitis + vaso-occlusion (young smoker)

Sx: Claudication, gangrene

PE:

Dx:

_____   Tx:

_____

_____

Raynaud's: Arteriole vasospasm

Sx: White, blue, red fingers

PE:

Dx:

RAYNAUDS PHENOMENON

WHITE DUE TO LACK OF BLOOD FLOW | PURPLE DUE TO LACK OF OXYGEN | RED WHEN BLOOD FLOW RETURNS

_____

_____

_____

Tx:

Varicose Veins: Great saphenous vein most commonly affected

Sx: Dilated, tortuous veins, pain with standing, edema

PE:

Dx:

_____   Tx:

_____

_____

Venous Insufficiency: **Stasis dermatitis**

Sx: Red/brown pigmented ulcers @ medial malleolus

PE:

Dx: US to rule out DVT

_____   **Tx:**

_____

_____

Carotid Occlusive Disease: **Atherosclerotic plaques**

Sx: Bruit, TIA

PE:

Dx: US, angiography

_____   **Tx:**

_____

_____

Hypertension, Cardiomyopathy, Heart Failure

Essential Hypertension:

Sx: Often asymptomatic

PE: Normal: Elevated:

     Stage 1:   Stage 2:

Dx: Labs:

    UA:

    EKG:

_____   Tx:

_____

_____

JNC Treatment Targets:

ASCVD Risk Calculator:

Secondary Hypertension: Can be due to kidney disease, endocrine disorders, cardiac issues, sleep apnea, obesity, medications, etc.

Risk Factors:

Sx:

PE: Elevated BP

Dx:

_____   Tx:

_____

_____

Hypertensive Urgency: > 180/120 without end-organ damage

Sx: May be asymptomatic, often will have headache

PE:

Dx:

_____   Tx:

_____

_____

Hypertensive Emergency: > 180/120 with end-organ damage

Sx: Neurological symptoms, nausea, vomiting

PE: Fundoscopic changes

Dx:

_____   Tx:

_____

_____

Malignant Hypertension (Hypertensive Crisis): Rapid elevation in BP with poor prognosis

Sx:

PE: Papilledema, encephalopathy, nephropathy, & A/V nicking

Dx:

_____   Tx:

_____

_____

Hypotension

Cardiogenic Shock:

Sx: Hypotension, tachycardia, tachypnea

PE:

Dx:

_____

_____

_____

Tx:

Orthostatic Hypotension:

Sx: Can be asymptomatic or experience dizziness, lightheadedness, and/or syncope

PE:

Dx:

_____

_____

_____

Tx:

Vasovagal Syncope: **Most common cause of syncope**

Sx: Hypotension, bradycardia, syncope with vagal maneuvers

PE:

Dx:

_____

_____

_____

Tx:

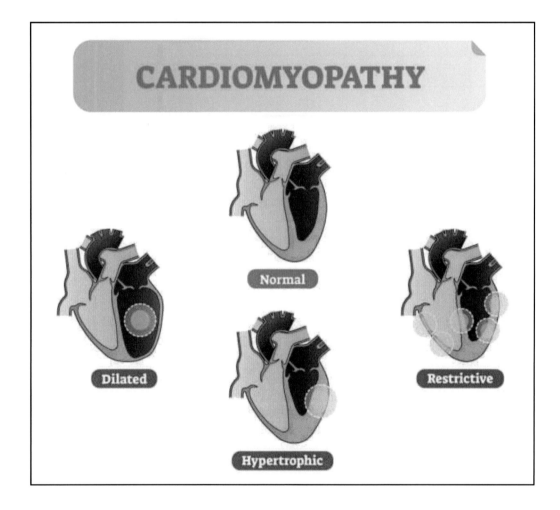

Dilated Cardiomyopathy: Enlargement primarily of left ventricle, with decreased wall thickness
All 4 chambers may be dilated in late stages
Causes: CAD, viral, EtOH, cocaine, OSA

Sx:

PE: S3, rales, JVD

Dx: Low ejection fraction < 50%

_____   Tx:

_____

_____

Hypertrophic Cardiomyopathy: Thick LV (commonly septum), impaired outflow, sudden death in athlete

Sx: SOB, palpitations, syncope, family history

Murmur:

Dx:

_____   Tx:

_____

_____

Restrictive Cardiomyopathy: Diastole, filling problem, normal ejection fraction
Associated with sarcoid and amyloidosis

Sx:

PE: S4, Kussmaul

Dx: Biopsy

_____   Tx:

_____

_____

Left Ventricular Systolic Heart Failure: (Pumping issue)

Sx: Tachycardia, narrow pulse pressure, diaphoresis, vasoconstriction

PE:

Dx: Ejection fraction < 40%, BNP > 400

_____   **Tx:**

_____

_____

Left Ventricular Diastolic Heart Failure: (Filling issue)

Sx: Heart failure symptoms

PE:

Dx: Normal ejection fraction

_____   **Tx:**

_____

_____

Right Heart Failure: Blood backups into the body

Sx: Edema, JVD, ascites

PE:

Dx:

_____   **Tx:**

_____

_____

Congenital Heart Defects

Atrial Septal Defect:

Sx:

Murmur:

Dx: EKG = RBBB

_____   Tx:

_____

_____

Ventricular Septal Defect:

Sx:

Murmur:

Dx: EKG, Chest X-ray, transthoracic echocardiogram

_____   Tx:

_____

_____

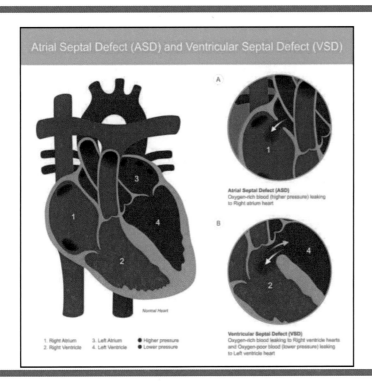

Atrial Septal Defect (ASD) and Ventricular Septal Defect (VSD)

Coarctation of Aorta: **Narrowing of aorta**

Sx:

PE: Asymmetric BP/pulse

Dx: Rib notching on Chest X-ray

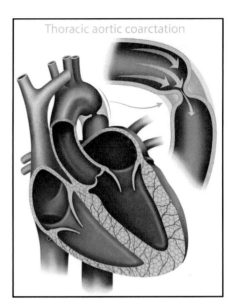

_____

_____

_____

Tx:

Patent Ductus Arteriosus: **Should close in 1st week of life, failure to thrive**

Sx: Bounding arterial pulse, cyanosis

Murmur:

Dx: EKG, echocardiogram

_____   Tx:

_____

_____

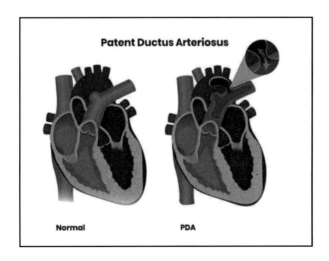

Tetralogy of Fallot: **Left to right shunting**

Sx: TET spells

Murmur:

Dx: Chest X-ray = boot shaped heart, left to right shunting

_____   **Tx:**

_____

_____

Normal heart   Tetralogy of Fallot

Atrial Myxoma: **Benign, rare cardiac tumor**

Sx:

PE:

Dx: Echocardiogram, EKG, Chest X-ray

_____   **Tx:**

_____

_____

Lipid Disorders

Hypercholesterolemia: Elevated total cholesterol, LDL, triglycerides - can be hereditary

Sx: Asymptomatic, xanthelasma

PE:

Dx: Hereditary = genetic testing

Labs = total cholesterol > 200, LDL > 100-130, HDL < 45

_____   Tx:

_____

_____

Hypertriglyceridemia:

Sx:

PE:

Dx: Labs = triglycerides > 150

_____   Tx:

_____

_____

Hypertension Medications

Alpha Blocker	Beta Blockers "olol"
Alpha 1	Beta 1- (crosses blood brain barrier)

Indications:

Indications:

SE:

SE:

Alpha 2 agonist

Indications:

SE:

```
Black Box Warning
```

ACE Inhibitors "pril"	ARB "sartan" (young, white)	Renin Inhibitor
Indications:	Indications:	Indications:
SE:	SE:	SE:

Black Box Warning

Calcium Channel Blocker: First line for black people & elderly - works on smooth muscle/visceral organs

Non-Dihydropyridines:	Dihydropyridines: "dipines"
Indications:	Indications:
SE:	SE:

Black Box Warning

Direct Acting Vasodilators

Indications:

SE:

Nitrates

Indications:

SE:

Diuretic

Early Distal Tubule	Loop of Henley	Far Distal Tubule
Thiazides: K+ wasting	**Loops:**	**K-sparing:**
Indications:	Indications:	Indications:
SE:	SE:	SE:

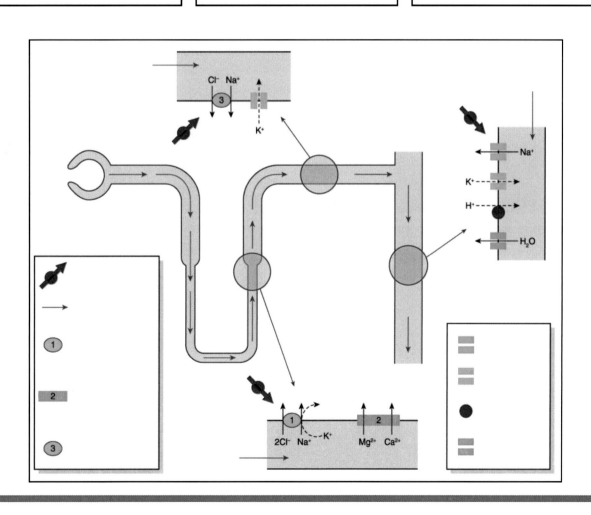

Anticoagulation

Vitamin K (Reversal) - PT/INR   **Heparins - PT**

Indications: Indications:

SE: SE:

> Heparin Induced Thrombocytopenia (HIT) – PE or DVT

Direct Oral Anticoagulants - DOAC (also called NOAC - Novel Oral Anticoagulants)

Indications:

SE:

Anti-Platelets - Inhibits thrombus formation

TxA2   P2Y12   Aspirin   Cox   PDE III

Indications:

SE:

Clotting Cascade

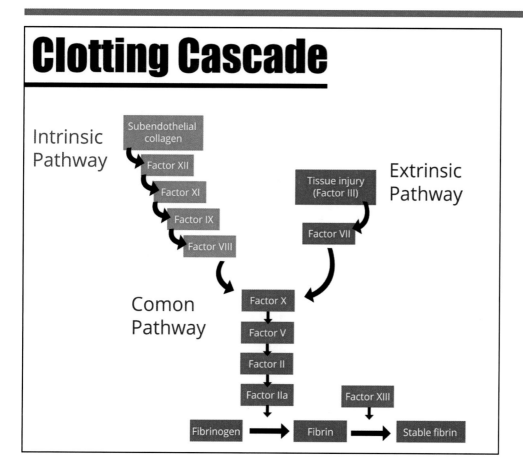

Intrinsic Pathway

Subendothelial collagen

Factor XII

Factor XI

Factor IX

Factor VIII

Tissue injury (Factor III)

Extrinsic Pathway

Factor VII

Comon Pathway

Factor X

Factor V

Factor II

Factor IIa

Factor XIII

Fibrinogen → Fibrin → Stable fibrin

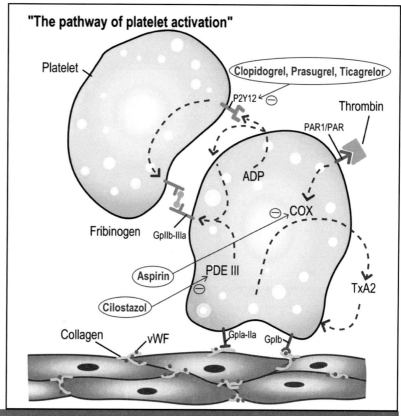

"The pathway of platelet activation"

Hypercholesterolemia Medications

Statins: Reduce cholesterol synthesis   SE:
Indications:

_____

_____

_____

PCSK9 Inhibitors   SE:
Indications:

_____

_____

_____

Bile Acid Sequestrants: SE:
Indications:

_____

_____

_____

Niacin: SE:
Indications:

_____

_____

_____

Ezetimibe: SE:
Indications:

_____

_____

_____

Fibrates: Lower triglycerides   SE:
Indications:

_____

_____

_____

Medications

_____ : MOA = _____

Indication(s) = _____

Side Effects = _____

Types/ Examples = _____

_____

_____

_____ : MOA = _____

Indication(s) = _____

Side Effects = _____

Types/ Examples = _____

_____

_____

_____ : MOA = _____

Indication(s) = _____

Side Effects = _____

Types/ Examples = _____

_____

_____

_____ : MOA = _____

Indication(s) = _____

Side Effects = _____

Types/ Examples = _____

_____

_____

_____ : MOA = _____

Indication(s) = _____

Side Effects = _____

Types/ Examples = _____

_____

Medications

_____: MOA = _____

Indication(s) = _____

Side Effects = _____

Types/ Examples = _____

_____

_____

_____: MOA = _____

Indication(s) = _____

Side Effects = _____

Types/ Examples = _____

_____

_____

_____: MOA = _____

Indication(s) = _____

Side Effects = _____

Types/ Examples = _____

_____

_____

_____: MOA = _____

Indication(s) = _____

Side Effects = _____

Types/ Examples = _____

_____

_____

_____: MOA = _____

Indication(s) = _____

Side Effects = _____

Types/ Examples = _____

_____

Pulmonology

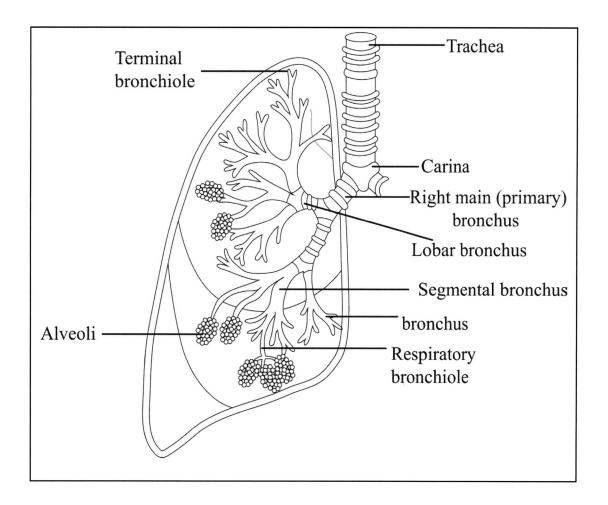

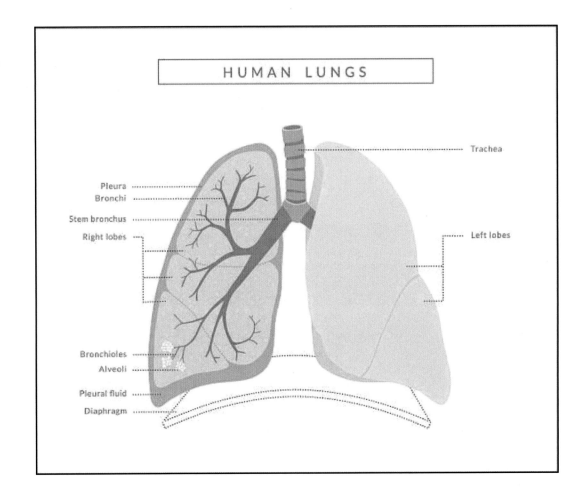

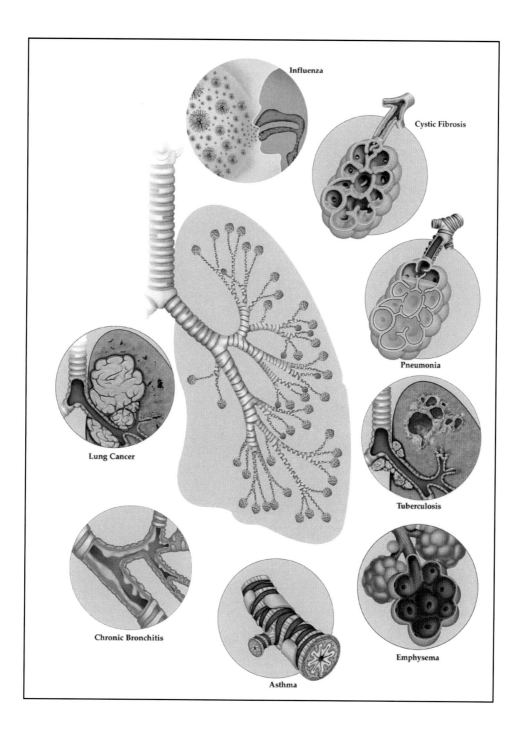

Influenza

Cystic Fibrosis

Pneumonia

Lung Cancer

Tuberculosis

Chronic Bronchitis

Asthma

Emphysema

Chronic Obstructive Pulmonary Disease:

Risk Factors:

1. Chronic Bronchitis 85%:

Sx: Chronic cough, productive sputum, dyspnea, prolonged expiration

PE: Rales, rhonchi, wheezing "Blue Bloaters"

2. Emphysema 15%:

Sx: Dyspnea, chronic cough (with or without sputum)

PE: Decreased breath sounds, barrel chest, hyperresonance, wheezing "Pink Puffer"

Dx: Tx:

_____

_____

_____

GOLD COPD Guidelines

Asthma:

Sx: Cough (more common at night), wheeze, shortness of breath

PE:

Dx: Low FEV1/FVC, normal DLCO

_____   Tx:

_____

_____

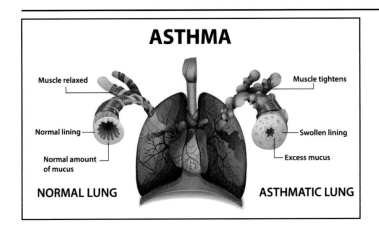

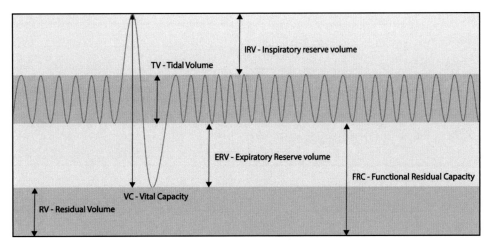

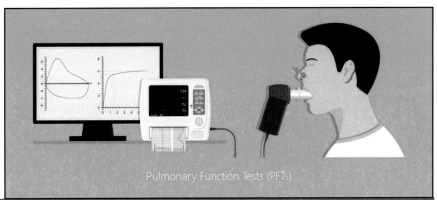

Obstructive Airway Medications

Beta 2 Agonist:

MOA = _____

Indication(s) = _____

Side Effects = _____

Types/ Examples = _____

_____

_____

Short Acting Beta Agonist (SABA):

MOA = _____

Indication(s) = _____

Side Effects = _____

Types/ Examples = _____

_____

_____

Long Acting Muscarinic Agonist (LAMA):

MOA = _____

Indication(s) = _____

Side Effects = _____

Types/ Examples = _____

_____

_____

Short Acting Muscarinic Agonist (SAMA):

MOA = _____

Indication(s) = _____

Side Effects = _____

Types/ Examples = _____

_____

_____

Inhaled Corticosteroids (ICS):

MOA = _____

Indication(s) = _____

Side Effects = _____

Types/ Examples = _____

_____

_____

Oral Glucocorticoid:

MOA = _____

Indication(s) = _____

Side Effects = _____

Types/ Examples = _____

_____

_____

Omalizumab:

MOA = _____

Indication(s) = _____

Side Effects = _____

Types/ Examples = _____

_____

_____

Mast Cell Stabilizers:

MOA = _____

Indication(s) = _____

Side Effects = _____

Types/ Examples = _____

_____

_____

Antileukotrienes:

MOA = _____

Indication(s) = _____

Side Effects = _____

Types/ Examples = _____

_____

_____

Antimuscarinics:

MOA = _____

Indication(s) = _____

Side Effects = _____

Types/ Examples = _____

_____

_____

Asthma management chart

Restrictive Pulmonary Disease

Restrictive pattern = normal or increased FEV 1/FVC, normal or decreased FVC, decreased lung volumes (VC, RV, FRC, TLC) decreased DLCO

Idiopathic Pulmonary Fibrosis: Progressive scarring of the lungs for unknown reasons

Sx:

PX: Fine, dry, bibasilar inspiratory crackles, clubbing

Dx:

_____   Tx:

_____

_____

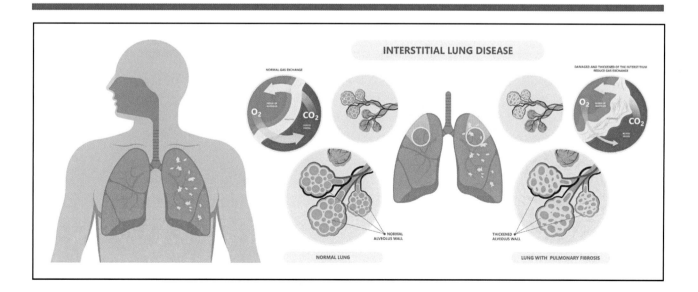

Pneumoconiosis

Asbestosis: Diffuse, progressive pulmonary fibrosis

Risk Factors:

Sx:

PE: Clubbing, bibasilar crackles

Dx:

_____   Tx:

_____

_____

Silicosis: Inhalation of silicon dioxide (coal mining, granite, slate, quartz, sandblasting, stone mason)

Sx: Chronic:

    Acute:

PE: Crackles

Dx:

_____   Tx:

_____

_____

Berylliosis: Granulomatous pulmonary disease caused by beryllium exposure

Risk Factors:

Sx: Dyspnea, cough, fever, weight loss

PE:

Dx:

_____   Tx:

_____

_____

Coal Worker's Pneumoconiosis (Black Lung): Inhalation of coal dust

Sx:

PX: Crackles

Dx:

_____

_____

_____

Tx:

Sarcoidosis:

Risk Factors: Females, African Americans, Northern Europeans

Sx:

PE: Lupus perino (specific), erythema nodosum (most common)

Dx: Bronchoscopy = gold standard

_____

_____

_____

Tx:

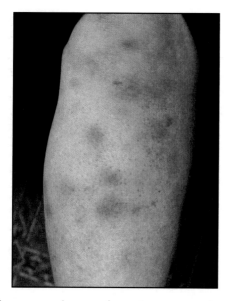

Erythema nodosum (most common)

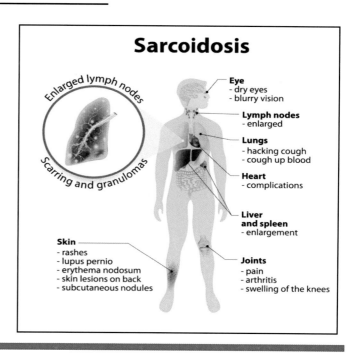

Infectious Pulmonary Disorders

Acute Bronchiolitis (RSV - Respiratory Syncytial Virus): Lower respiratory tract

Sx: Cough, fever, wheeze

PE:

Dx:

_____   Tx:

_____

_____

Acute Bronchitis: Most common is viral

Sx: Cough 5-21 days, #1 cause of hemoptysis

PE:

Dx:

_____

_____

_____

Tx:

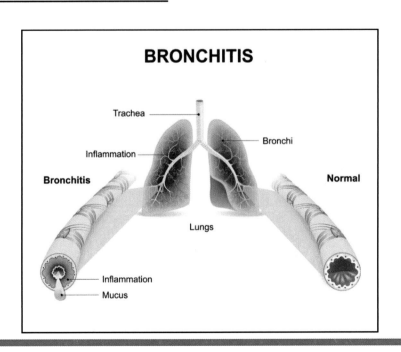

Pertussis "Whooping Cough": Bordetella pertussis - gram neg rod

3 stages:

Sx: Inspiratory stridor/whoop, emesis, fever

PE:

Dx: X-ray = perihilar infiltrates, atelectasis

_____ **Tx:**

_____

_____

Vaccine:

Influenza A&B:

Sx: Fever, sore throat, cough, lymphadenopathy

PE:

Dx: Clinical, viral culture or rapid antigen test

_____ **Tx:**

_____

_____

Pneumonia:

Complications: Empyema, abscess

Sx: Productive cough, rales, decreased breath sounds, fever + WBC + infiltrate

PE:

Dx:

_____   Tx:

_____

_____

Vaccine:

CURB 65

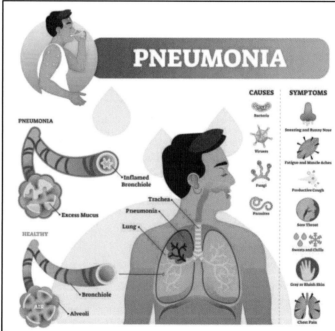

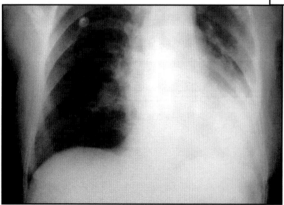

Bacterial Pneumonia

Pneumococcal Pneumonia: Strep pneumoniae (gram-positive diplococci), community acquired pneumonia (CAP)

Sx: Rust sputum

Dx: Tx:

M. Catarrhalis: COPD, elderly

Sx: Systemic symptoms

Dx: Tx:

Haemophilus Influenzae: Gram negative - second most common cause of CAP

Sx: Meningitis symptoms but no rash, HIB meningitis - seen in babies 6-24 months

Dx: Clinical, physical exam   Tx:

Atypical Pneumonia

Chlamydia Pneumoniae: College kids, sore throat

Sx: Cough, fever, rales

Dx: Tx:

Legionella: Air conditioning, water source

Sx: Fever, headache, crackles/rhonchi, hyponatremia, diarrhea

Dx: Tx:

Mycoplasma Pneumoniae: "Walking pneumonia", school aged children, college students, military

Sx:

Dx: X-ray = reticulonodular pattern, PCR, serology, cold agglutination   Tx:

Healthcare Acquired Pneumonia

Causes: IV wound care, hospitalized within 90 days, outpatient treatment in hospital (i.e., dialysis)

Pseudomonas: Green sputum

Sx:

Dx: X-ray = progressive infiltrates   Tx:

Other Pneumonia

Aspiration Pneumonia: Strep, staph, haemophilus influenzae, klebsiella, and anaerobes

Sx: Cough, dyspnea, fever, pleuritic chest pain

Dx: Tx:

Viral Pneumonia: Inflammation of alveolar walls

Most Common Cause: Kids = RSV

Adults = influenza A & B, Covid

Sx: Afebrile

Dx: X-ray = diffuse infiltrates   Tx:

Tuberculosis: **Mycobacterium**

Sx: Hemoptysis, weight loss, night sweats, fever

PE:

Dx: Latent Dx:

    Active Dx:

_____   **Tx:**

TB testing:

    PPD -

    QuantiFERON Gold -

    Chest X-ray -

Vaccine:

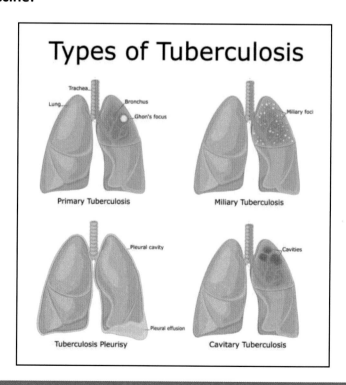

Bronchiectasis: Permanent dilation and destruction of the airway, most common cause is cystic fibrosis

Sx: Chronic cough, *foul smelling sputum*, hemoptysis, clubbing, recurrent pneumonia

PE: Crackles, wheezing, rhonchi

Dx:

_____

_____

_____

Tx:

BRONCHIECTASIS
(obstructive lung disease)

Lung Abscess: Anaerobes, seen in alcoholics and those with epilepsy, most common in right lower lobe

Sx: Cough, fever, chills, purulent sputum

PE:

Dx:

_____

_____

_____

Tx:

Lung Abscess

Empyema: Purulent fluid in pleural space

Sx: Persistent fever, recent pneumonia, constitutional symptoms

PE:

Dx:

_____

_____

_____

Tx:

Pulmonic Nodules and Neoplasms

Small Cell Lung Cancer: Smoking #1 cause, aggressive

Sx: Hemoptysis, dyspnea, asymptomatic

PE:

Dx:

_____   Tx:

_____

_____

Squamous Cell Lung Cancer: Non-small cell lung cancer, smoking

Sx: Hemoptysis, dyspnea, asymptomatic

PE:

Dx:

_____   Tx:

_____

_____

Large Cell Lung Cancer:

Sx: Pleuritic pain, dyspnea, cough

PE:

Dx:

_____   Tx:

_____

_____

Adenocarcinoma: **Non-smokers**

Sx: Pleuritic pain, dyspnea, cough

PE:

Dx:

_____   **Tx:**

_____

_____

Pulmonary Nodules:

Sx: Can be asymptomatic, dyspnea, cough

PE: Round lesion that is > 3cm and surrounded by lung parenchyma

Dx:

_____   **Tx:**

_____

_____

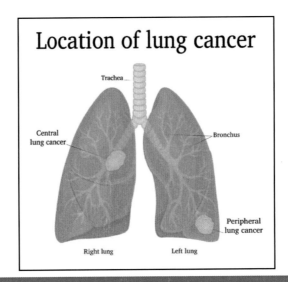

Pleural Diseases

Pleural Effusions: Fluid in pleural space

Sx:

PE:

Dx: X-ray, CT, thoracentesis

_____

_____

_____

Pleural fluid analysis = Light's Criteria
  Gram stain/culture
        Transudate: More likely bilateral
        Exudate: More likely unilateral high protein, high LDH

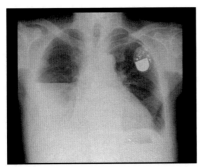

Tx: Depends on underlying cause

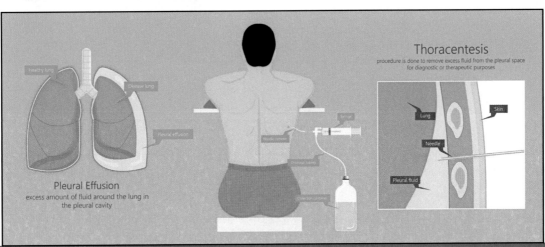

Pneumothorax: **Air in pleural space**

Sx: Acute chest pain, shortness of breath, decreased breath sounds, hyperresonance
   Spontaneous=
   Tension=

PE:

Dx:

_____

_____

_____

Tx: Small:

   Large:

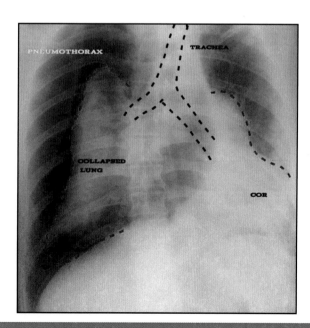

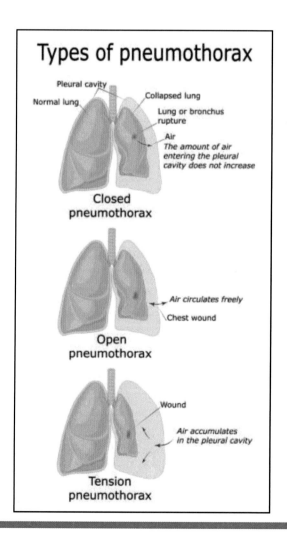

Pulmonary Circulation Disorders

Pulmonary Embolism:

Risk Factor:

Sx:

PE: Virchow's Triad:

Dx: CTA pulmonary angiogram = gold standard

    X-ray:

    EKG:

_____

_____

_____

Tx:

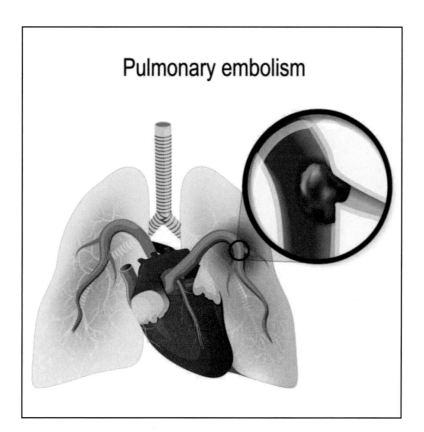

Pulmonary embolism

Pulmonary Hypertension: **Pulmonary artery pressure > 25 mmHg**

Sx: Right heart failure symptoms, shortness of breath, chest pain

PE:

Dx:

_____   Tx:

_____

_____

Primary/idiopathic: Tx:

Secondary: Tx:

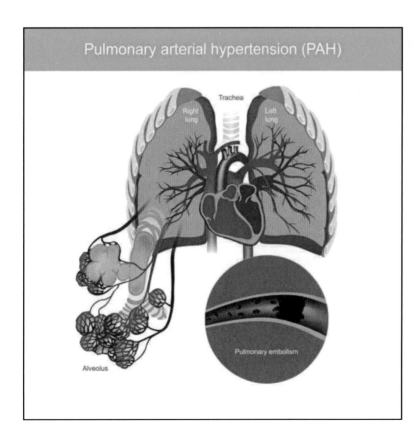

Sleep Apnea: **Obstructive or central**

Sx:

PE:

Dx: History, polysomnography

_____   Tx:

_____

_____

Other Pulmonary Disorders

Acute Respiratory Distress Syndrome - *EMERGENCY*

Known as Respiratory Distress Syndrome or "Hyaline Membrane Disease" in preterm infants. Low Surfactant

Sx:

PE:

Dx: X-ray:

   PaO2/FiO2: < 200

   Wedge pressure:

_____   Tx:

_____

_____

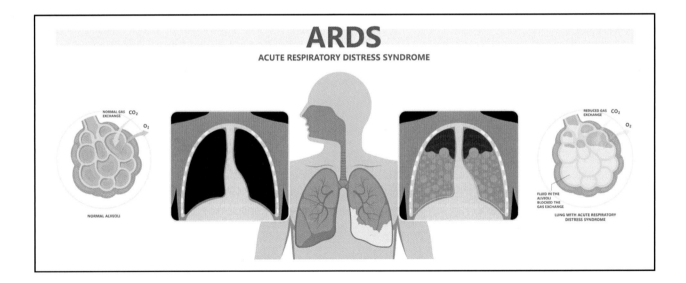

Samter's Triad:

Sx: Aspirin sensitivity + asthma + nasal polyps

PE:

Dx:

_____   Tx:

_____

_____

Cystic Fibrosis: Autosomal recessive

Sx:

PE: Nasal polyps, pancreatic insufficiency

Dx: Sweat chloride test

_____   Tx:

_____

_____

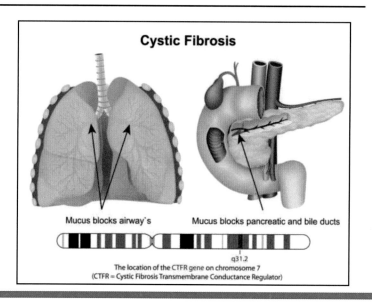

Cystic Fibrosis

Mucus blocks airway's

Mucus blocks pancreatic and bile ducts

q31.2
The location of the CTFR gene on chromosome 7
(CTFR = Cystic Fibrosis Transmembrane Conductance Regulator)

Foreign Body Aspiration: **Most common right side**

Sx: Stridor, cough, wheezing

PE:

Dx: X-ray can be normal, bronchoscopy

_____   **Tx:**

_____

_____

Atelectasis: **Alveolar collapse, can be full or partial**

Sx: Trouble breathing, cough, chest pain

PE:

Dx: X-ray

_____   **Tx:**

_____

_____

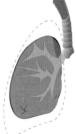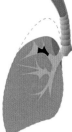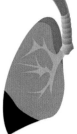

Atelectasis

Contraction atelectasis   Resorption atelectasis   Compression atelectasis

Obesity Hypoventilation Syndrome:

Sx: Daytime sleepiness, fatigue, impaired memory

PE: Obese body habitus

Dx:

---

*Acute Epiglottitis: **In EENT***

*Croup (Parainfluenza): **In EENT***

Medications

_____ : MOA = _____

Indication(s)=_____

Side Effects = _____

Types/ Examples = _____

_____

_____

_____ : MOA = _____

Indication(s)=_____

Side Effects = _____

Types/ Examples = _____

_____

_____

_____ : MOA = _____

Indication(s)=_____

Side Effects = _____

Types/ Examples = _____

_____

_____

_____ : MOA = _____

Indication(s)=_____

Side Effects = _____

Types/ Examples = _____

_____

_____

_____ : MOA = _____

Indication(s)=_____

Side Effects = _____

Types/ Examples = _____

_____

Medications

_____: MOA = _____

Indication(s)=_____

Side Effects = _____

Types/ Examples = _____

_____

_____

_____: MOA = _____

Indication(s)=_____

Side Effects = _____

Types/ Examples = _____

_____

_____

_____: MOA = _____

Indication(s)=_____

Side Effects = _____

Types/ Examples = _____

_____

_____

_____: MOA = _____

Indication(s)=_____

Side Effects = _____

Types/ Examples = _____

_____

_____

_____: MOA = _____

Indication(s)=_____

Side Effects = _____

Types/ Examples = _____

_____

Gastrointestinal Disorders

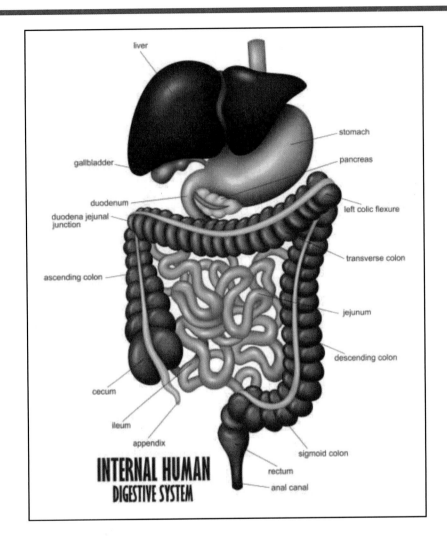

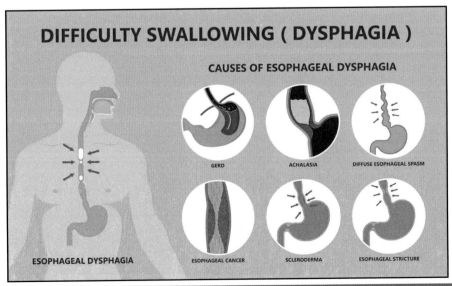

Esophageal Disorders

Eosinophilic Esophagitis: Eosinophilic infiltration of esophageal tissue

Sx:

PE:

Dx: Endoscopy +/- corrugated rings

_____   **Tx:**

_____

_____

Pill Induced Esophagitis:

Sx: Painful swallowing, dysphagia

PE:

Dx:

_____   **Tx:**

_____

_____

Infectious Esophagitis: Seen in immunocompromised patients

Sx: Candida = white plaques

    EBV, TB, MAC, CMV = large ulcers

    HSV = punched lesions

PE:

Dx:

_____   **Tx:**

_____

_____

Non-Infectious Esophagitis: GERD most common etiology

Sx: Painful swallowing, heartburn, dysphagia, belching

PE:

Dx:

_____

_____

_____

Tx:

Gastroesophageal Reflux Disease (GERD): Can lead to Barrett's esophagus

Sx:

PE:

Dx: EGD

_____

_____

_____

Gastroesophageal reflux disease

Esophagus
Sphincter closed
Stomach
Healthy

Sphincter open, allowing reflux
GERD

Tx:

Barrett's Esophagus: Precancerous metaplastic columnar cells

Sx:

PE:

Dx: Endoscopy with biopsy

_____

_____

_____

Tx:

Mallory-Weiss Tear: **Tear in mucosa - most commonly from vomiting**

Sx:

PE:

Dx: EGD

_____   Tx:

_____

_____

Achalasia:

Sx: Dysphagia of both solids and liquids

PE:

Dx: Swallow study with bird beak, manometry > 45mmHg

_____

_____

_____

Tx:

Diffuse Esophageal Spasms (DES):

Sx:

PE:

Dx: Barium swallow with corkscrew, manometry

_____   Tx:

_____

_____

Nutcracker Esophagus: **Severe DES**

Sx:

PE:

Dx: Manometry > 180 mmHg

_____   **Tx:**

_____

_____

Esophageal Strictures:

Sx: Dysphagia with solid foods

PE:

Dx: Endoscopy

_____   **Tx:**

_____

_____

Esophageal (Schatzki) Ring: **Most commonly associated with sliding hiatal hernia**

Sx:

PE:

Dx: Barium esophagram

_____   **Tx:**

_____

_____

Esophageal Varices: **Portal hypertension**

Sx:

PE:

Dx: Upper endoscopy

_____

_____

_____

Tx:

Esophageal Varices

Esophageal varices

Esophagus — Liver with cirrhosis

Portal vein

Stomach

Boerhaave's: **Esophageal rupture/perforation**

Sx:

PE:

Dx: Chest X-ray (initial), CT, contrast esophagram (diagnostic)

_____   Tx:

_____

_____

Zenker's Diverticulum: **Pharyngeal pouch**

Sx: Foul odor

PE:

Dx: Barium swallow

_____   Tx:

_____

_____

Gastric Disorders

Gastritis: Causes - H. pylori, autoimmune, NSAIDs

Sx:

PE:

Dx: EGD with biopsy

_____

_____

_____

Tx:

DISEASES OF THE STOMACH

Gastric ulcer

Gastritis
Inflammation of the gastric mucosa

Peptic Ulcer Disease: Causes - H. pylori, medications, Zollinger-Ellison

Sx:

PE:

Dx: Endoscopy (Gold Standard) +/- biopsy

_____

_____

_____

Tx:

Location of peptic ulcer

ESOPHAGUS

Esophageal ulcer

Duodenal ulcer

Gastric ulcer

STOMACH

DUODENUM

H. Pylori: Gram-negative bacteria

Sx:

PE:

Dx: Urea breath test, fecal antigen test, blood work

_____

_____

_____

Tx:

HELICOBACTER PYLORI

Zollinger-Ellison Syndrome: **Neuroendocrine tumor that secretes gastrin**

Sx:

PE:

Dx: High gastrin levels

_____

_____

_____

Tx:

Pyloric Stenosis: **Males aged 3-6 weeks**

Sx:

PE: RUQ mass - olive shaped

Dx:

_____   Tx:

_____

_____

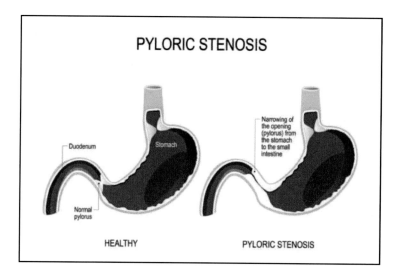

PYLORIC STENOSIS

Duodenum
Stomach
Normal pylorus

Narrowing of the opening (pylorus) from the stomach to the small intestine

HEALTHY   PYLORIC STENOSIS

Biliary Disorders

Cholecystitis:

Risk Factors: Female, fat, forty, fertile

Sx:

PE: + Murphy's sign

Dx: HIDA gold standard

_____

_____

_____

Tx:

Cholelithiasis:

Sx: Colicky RUQ pain

PE:

Dx: US

_____

_____

_____

Tx:

Choledocholithiasis: Common bile duct obstruction

Sx:

PE:

Dx: ERCP

_____

_____

_____

Tx:

Acute Ascending Cholangitis: **Infection of biliary tree**

Sx: Charcot's triad:

    Reynold's pentad:

PE:

Dx: ERCP

_____

_____

_____

Tx:

Primary Sclerosis Cholangitis: **Chronic inflammation of liver and bile ducts**

Sx:

PE:

Dx: ERCP

_____

_____

_____

Tx:

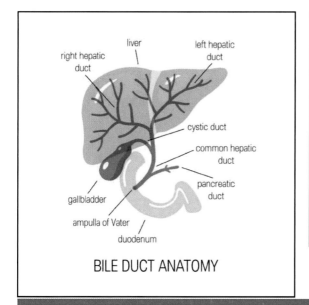

BILE DUCT ANATOMY

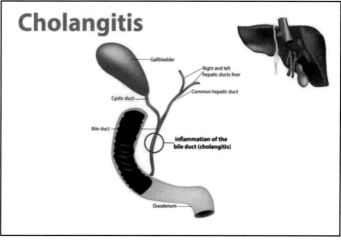

Hepatitis A: **Fecal-oral**

Sx:

PE:

Dx: Anti-HAV IgM

_____   **Tx:**

_____

_____

Hepatitis B:

Sx:

PE:

Dx: Vaccinated: + Anti-HBs

Acute inf: +HBsAg +/- antiHBc IgM

Chronic: + HBsAg + Anti-HBc IgG HBeAg = infective

_____

_____

_____

Hepatitis C: **Blood borne**

Sx:

PE:

Dx: HCV Ab

_____   **Tx:**

_____

_____

The PA Bible

Hepatitis A: **Fecal-oral**

Sx:

PE:

Dx: Anti-HAV IgM

Tx:

Hepatitis B:

Sx:

PE:

Dx: Vaccinated: + Anti-HBs

Acute inf: +HBsAg +/- antiHBc IgM

Chronic: + HBsAg + Anti-HBc IgG HBeAg = infective

Hepatitis C: **Blood borne**

Sx:

PE:

Dx: HCV Ab

Tx:

98

Hepatitis D: **Only occurs with Hepatitis B**

Sx:

PE:

Dx:

_____   Tx:

_____

_____

Hepatitis E: **Fecal-oral**

Sx:

PE:

Dx: IgM anti-HEV

_____   Tx:

_____

_____

Autoimmune Hepatitis:

Sx: Fatigue, anorexia, abdominal pain, hepatomegaly, jaundice

PE:

Dx:

_____   Tx:

_____

_____

Cirrhosis:

Sx:

PE: Ascites, caput medusa, encephalopathy

Dx: US

_____   **Tx:**

_____

_____

Fatty Liver Disease: Commonly associated with obesity, dyslipidemia, diabetes, and alcohol

Sx:

PE:

Dx:

_____   **Tx:**

_____

_____

Budd-Chiari Syndrome:

Sx: Abdominal pain esophageal varices, ascites

PE:

Dx:

_____   Tx:

_____

_____

Gilbert's: Inherited disorder leading to impaired conjugation of biliribin

Sx: Episodic jaundice with stress

PE:

Dx:

_____   Tx:

_____

_____

Primary Biliary Cholangitis: Immunologic attack

Sx: Itching, jaundice, xanthelasma

PE:

Dx:

_____   Tx:

_____

_____

Pancreatic & Small Bowel Disorders

Pancreatitis:

Sx: Epigastric pain that radiates to the back

PE: Grey Turner's & Cullen's sign

Dx: Ranson's Criteria

_____   Tx:

_____

_____

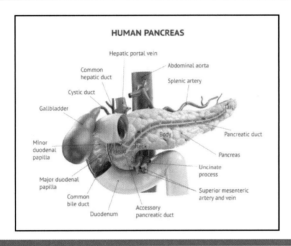

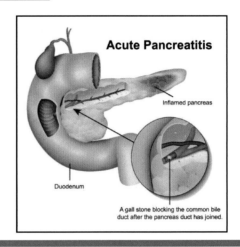

Appendicitis: Most common cause is fecalith

Sx: RLQ pain

PE: McBurney's, Rovsing sign, Obturator, Psoas

Dx:

_____

_____

_____

Tx:

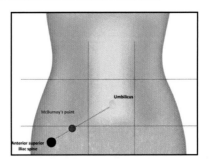

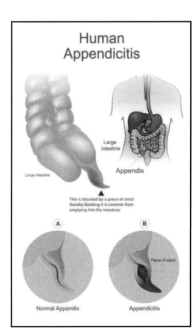

Bowel Obstruction:

Small bowel obstruction: **Post-op adhesions, high pitched bowel sounds**

_____   Tx:

_____

_____

Large bowel obstruction: **Impaction, tumor**

_____   Tx:

_____

_____

Dx:

Paralytic Ileus (Ogilvie's): **Pseudo-obstructions, decreased peristalsis without obstruction**

Sx:

PE:

Dx:

_____   Tx:

_____

_____

Ischemic Colitis:

Sx:

PE: Severe abdominal pain with bloody diarrhea

Dx: Colonoscopy

_____   **Tx:**

_____

_____

Volvulus:

Sigmoid (elderly)

Midgut (infants)

Sx:

PE:

Dx: X-ray = coffee bean

       CT = whirlpool/twist

VOLVULUS OF THE COLON

Sigmoid colon   Volvulus

180°

Fulcrum for the twist

_____   **Tx:**

_____

_____

Colorectal Disorders

Anorectal Abscess:

Sx:

PE:

Dx: Clinical

_____   Tx:

_____

_____

Anorectal Fistula: Complication of deep abscess

Risk Factor: Crohn's

Sx: Anal discharge and pain

PE:

Dx:

FISTULAS OF THE RECTUM

_____

_____

_____

Tx:

Anal Fissure: Tear distal to dentate line - most commonly posterior

Sx: Rectal pain with bowel movement

PE:

Dx:

Cross section of rectum & anus

_____

_____

_____

Tx:

Constipation: < 2 weeks, most common causes = opiates, hypothyroidism, dehydration

Sx:

PE:

Dx:

_____   Tx:

_____

_____

Hemorrhoids: **Engorged rectal veins**

Sx: Internal = nonpainful, bleeding, pruritis

    External = painful

PE:

Dx:

_____

_____

_____

Tx:

Colon Polyps:

Sx: Often asymptomatic

PE:

Dx: Colonoscopy with biopsy

_____

_____

_____

Tx:

Lynch Syndrome: Inherited disorder increasing risk of colon cancer

Sx:

PE:

Dx: Colonoscopy with biopsy

_____

_____

_____

Tx:

Peutz-Jeghers Syndrome: Autosomal dominant, hamartomatous polyps, hyperpigmentation (lips, oral mucosa, hands)

Sx:

PE:

Dx: Colonoscopy with biopsy

_____

_____

_____

Tx:

Diverticulosis: **Out pouching of colon mucosa**

Sx: Left lower quadrant colicky pain, painless rectal bleeding

PE:

Dx:

_____   **Tx:**

_____

_____

DIVERTICULOSIS and DIVERTICULITIS

Diverticulitis:

Sx: LLQ pain, fever

PE:

Dx: CT with fat stranding, leukocytosis

_____   **Tx:**

_____

_____

Intussusception: **Telescoping of intestines**

Sx: Intermittent abdominal pain, bloody stool

PE:

Dx:

_____   **Tx:**

_____

_____

Toxic Megacolon:

Sx: Fever, abdominal pain, nausea, vomiting, rectal bleeding, bloating

PE:

Dx:

_____

_____

_____

Tx:

Irritable Bowel Syndrome (IBS):

Sx:

PE:

Dx: Diagnosis of exclusion - ROME IV criteria

_____

_____

_____

Tx:

Inflammatory Bowel Disease:
Inflammatory, autoimmune

Ulcerative Colitis:

Sx: Bloody diarrhea, lower abdominal pain

PE:

Dx:

_____   Tx:

_____

_____

Risk for cancer & toxic megacolon

Inflammatory bowel disease (IBD)

Ulcerative colitis   Crohn's disease

Crohn's: Mouth to anus

Sx:

PE:

Dx: Cobblestoning, skip lesions

_____   Tx:

_____

_____

Risk for granuloma, fissure, fistulas

GI Neoplasms

Esophageal Cancer:

Sx: Dysphagia

PE:

Dx: EGD with biopsy

_____

_____

_____

Tx:

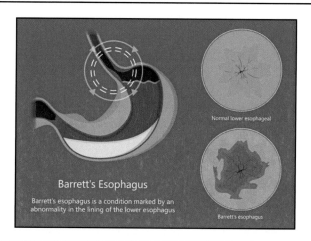

Adenocardinoma: Distal ⅓ - Barrett's esophagus precursor

Sx:

PE:

Dx:

_____   Tx:

_____

_____

Squamous Cell Carcinoma: **Proximal 2/3**

Sx:

PE:

Dx:

_____   **Tx:**

_____

_____

Stomach Cancer:

Risk Factors: H. pylori, salts, smoked meats, low fiber

Sx:

PE: Sister Mary Joseph nodule

Dx: EGD

Stomach cancer

_____

_____

_____

Tx:

Hepatocellular Carcinoma: **Most common in cirrhosis**

Sx:

PE:

Dx: Alpha-fetoprotein

_____   **Tx:**

_____

_____

Pancreatic Cancer: **Head of pancreas**

Sx:

PE: Courvoisier's (painless jaundice, palpable nontender gallbladder)

Dx: CT, CA 19-9

_____   Tx:

_____

_____

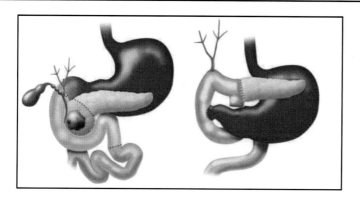

Colon Cancer: **Most common adenocarcinoma**

Sx: Painless rectal bleeding

PE:

Dx: Apple core lesion on barium enema, CEA

_____   Tx:

_____

_____

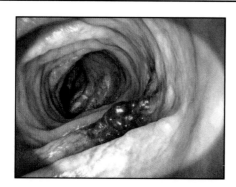

Carcinoid Syndrome: **MEN Type 1 (MEN1)**

Sx: Abdominal pain, weight loss, palpitations, diarrhea, flushing

PE:

Dx:

_____

_____

_____

Metabolic Disorders & Misc. GI

Phenylketonuria (PKU): Autosomal recessive

Sx: Mental retardation, odor

PE:

Dx:

_____

_____   Tx:

_____

Celiac: Autoimmune triggered by gluten, villous atrophy

Sx:

PE:

Dx: Anti-tissue transglutaminase

_____

_____

_____

Tx:

CELIAC DISEASE

HEALTHY INTESTINE

Normal villi

Small intestine

CELIAC DISEASE

Villous atrophy

Wilson's:

Sx: Dementia, cirrhosis, Kayser-Fleischer rings, Parkinson's

PE:

Dx: High free Cu, low total serum Cu

_____

_____

_____

Tx:

WILSON'S DISEASE

CNS disorders

Kayser-Fleischer ring

Hepatomegaly

Cardiomyopathy

Renal tubular dysfunction

Arthritis

Copper accumulates in tissues

Cu

Lactose Intolerance:

Sx:

PE:

Dx: Trial of lactose elimination

_____   Tx:

_____

_____

Hernias

Indirect Inguinal Hernia: Through internal inguinal ring - lateral

Sx:

PE:

Dx:

_____

_____

_____

Tx:

Inguinal Hernia

inferior epigastric vessels

direct

inguinal ligament

Hasselbach's

indirect

femoral

rectus abdominis muscle

Direct Inguinal Hernia: In external inguinal ring - medial

Sx:

PE:

Dx:

_____

_____

_____

Tx:

Hiatal/Diaphragmatic Hernia: Stomach through esophageal hiatus

Sx:

PE:

Dx:

TYPES OF HIATAL HERNIA

NORMAL ESOPHAGUS AND STOMACH

HIATAL HERNIA Type 1 (sliding)

HIATAL HERNIA Type 2 (rolling)

HIATAL HERNIA Type 3 (mixed)

_____

_____

_____

Tx:

Epigastric/Ventral Hernia: **Often at a surgical site**

Sx:

PE:

Dx:

_____   **Tx:**

_____

_____

Umbilical Hernia: **Seen at birth**

Sx:

PE:

Dx:

_____   **Tx:**

_____

_____

Femoral Hernia: **In femoral ring - risk of strangulation**

Sx:

PE:

Dx:

_____   **Tx:**

_____

_____

Diarrhea

Sx:

PE:

Dx:

S. Aureus: Picnic, egg salad

_____

Tx: _____

Vibrio Cholera: Shellfish

_____

Tx: _____

C. Perifringes: Canned food

_____

Tx: _____

Shigella: Daycare center, swimming, contaminated food

_____

Tx: _____

Salmonella: Meat, poultry, eggs, dairy

_____

Tx: _____

Rotavirus: Daycare center

_____

Tx: _____

Norovirus: Cruise ship

_____

Tx: _____

Giardia: Mountain water, foul stool

_____

Tx: _____

Traveler's Diarrhea: Most common E. coli

_____

Tx: _____

Typhoid:

_____

Tx: _____

Cholera:

_____

Tx: _____

Clostridium Difficile: Often associated with recent antibiotic use

Sx:

PE:

Dx: Stool culture

_____   Tx:

_____

_____

Bariatric Surgeries

Dumping Syndrome:

Sx:

PE:

Dx:

_____   Tx:

_____

_____

Vitamin Deficiencies

A: Night vision loss, dry skin, Bitot spots in eye

B1 (Thiamine): **Alcoholism, malnutrition, Wernicke-Korsakoff**

B2 (Riboflavin): **Glossitis, seborrheic dermatitis**

B3 (Niacin): **Dermatitis, dementia, diarrhea (Pellagra)**

B6 (Pyridoxine): **Sideroblastic anemia, weakness, insomnia, peripheral neuropathy**

B12 (Cobalamin): **Megaloblastic anemia + neurological symptoms**

C (Ascorbic acid): **Scurvy (bleeding, anemia, loose teeth)**

D: **Rickets (children), osteomalacia**

E: **Anemia, peripheral neuropathy, ataxia**

K: **Bleeding, PTT, normal bleeding time**

Vitamin Excess

A:

_____

_____

B3:

_____

_____

C:

_____

_____

D:

_____

_____

*Pilonidal Disease: **In Derm***

*G6PD Deficiency: **In Heme***

*Hemochromatosis: **In Heme***

Medications

_____: MOA = _____

Indication(s)=_____

Side Effects = _____

Types/ Examples = _____

_____

_____

_____: MOA = _____

Indication(s)=_____

Side Effects = _____

Types/ Examples = _____

_____

_____

_____: MOA = _____

Indication(s)=_____

Side Effects = _____

Types/ Examples = _____

_____

_____

_____: MOA = _____

Indication(s)=_____

Side Effects = _____

Types/ Examples = _____

_____

_____

_____: MOA = _____

Indication(s)=_____

Side Effects = _____

Types/ Examples = _____

_____

Medications

_____: MOA = _____

Indication(s)=_____

Side Effects = _____

Types/ Examples = _____

_____

_____

_____: MOA = _____

Indication(s)=_____

Side Effects = _____

Types/ Examples = _____

_____

_____

_____: MOA = _____

Indication(s)=_____

Side Effects = _____

Types/ Examples = _____

_____

_____

_____: MOA = _____

Indication(s)=_____

Side Effects = _____

Types/ Examples = _____

_____

_____

_____: MOA = _____

Indication(s)=_____

Side Effects = _____

Types/ Examples = _____

_____

Musculoskeletal/Ortho/Rheumatology

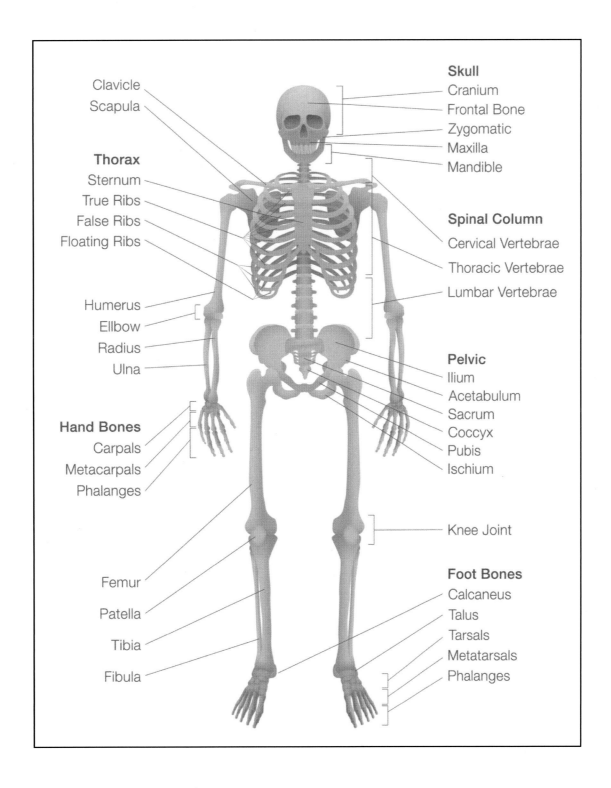

Clavicle
Scapula

Thorax
Sternum
True Ribs
False Ribs
Floating Ribs

Humerus
Ellbow
Radius
Ulna

Hand Bones
Carpals
Metacarpals
Phalanges

Femur
Patella
Tibia
Fibula

Skull
Cranium
Frontal Bone
Zygomatic
Maxilla
Mandible

Spinal Column
Cervical Vertebrae
Thoracic Vertebrae
Lumbar Vertebrae

Pelvic
Ilium
Acetabulum
Sacrum
Coccyx
Pubis
Ischium

Knee Joint

Foot Bones
Calcaneus
Talus
Tarsals
Metatarsals
Phalanges

HUMAN SKULL

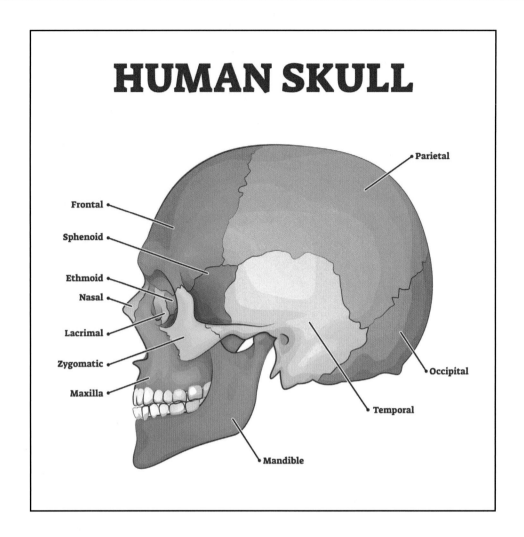

TYPES OF FRACTURE

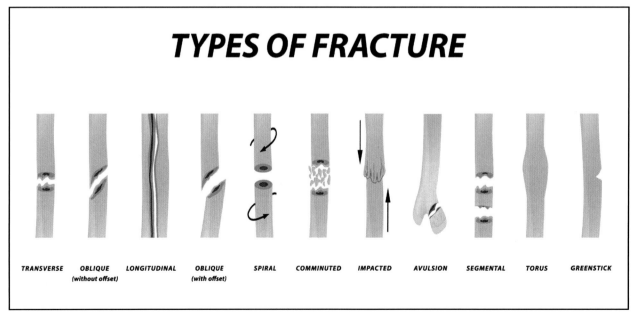

TRANSVERSE   OBLIQUE (without offset)   LONGITUDINAL   OBLIQUE (with offset)   SPIRAL   COMMINUTED   IMPACTED   AVULSION   SEGMENTAL   TORUS   GREENSTICK

Disorders of the Elbow & Forearm

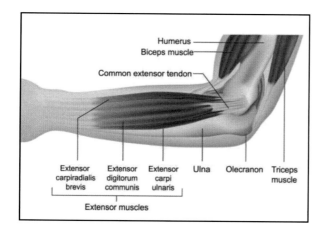

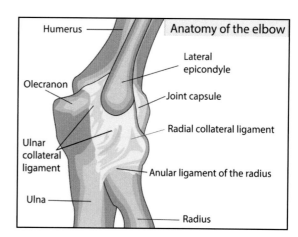

Elbow Dislocation: **Most common is posterior dislocation**

Sx: In flexion

PE:

Dx: X-ray

_____ Tx:

_____

_____

Olecranon Bursitis: **Swelling from overuse**

Sx: Pain at the site of the bursa

PE: Tenderness to palpation, decreased range of motion

Dx:

_____ Tx:

_____

_____

Biceps Tendonitis: **Caused from overuse**

Sx: Pain at bicipital groove

PE:

Dx: Yergason

_____   Tx:

_____

_____

Biceps Tendon Rupture: **Usually trauma**

Sx: Sudden sharp pain, sometimes a "pop" sound

PE: Popeye deformity

Dx:

_____

_____   Tx:

_____

Medial Epicondylitis: **Golfer's elbow**

Sx: Elbow pain during or following flexion

PE: Pain with resisted forearm pronation or wrist flexion

Dx:

_____   Tx:

_____

_____

Lateral Epicondylitis: **Tennis elbow**

Sx: Pain with extension

PE: Pain during resisted wrist and digit extension

Dx:

_____

_____   Tx:

_____

Elbow & Supracondylar Fractures:

Sx:

PX:

Dx: X-ray with anterior fat pad sign

    Sail sign = kids

    Radial head or proximal ulnar = adults

_____   **Tx:**

_____

_____

posterior sail sign   anterior sail sign

Radial Head Fracture: Most common in kids with FOOSH

Sx: Localized swelling, tender, decreased motion

PE:

Dx: X-ray

_____   **Tx:**

_____

_____

Nightstick Fracture: **Isolated fracture of ulna**

Sx:

PE:

Dx: X-ray

_____   Tx:

_____

_____

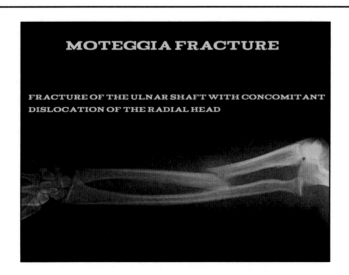

Monteggia Fracture: **Proximal ulnar fracture & radial head dislocation**

Sx: May have swelling, deformity, movement may cause pain

PE:

Dx: X-ray

_____   Tx:

_____

_____

MOTEGGIA FRACTURE

FRACTURE OF THE ULNAR SHAFT WITH CONCOMITANT
DISLOCATION OF THE RADIAL HEAD

Galeazzi Fracture: Distal radial fracture & radioulnar dislocation

Sx:

PX:

Dx: X-ray

_____

_____   Tx:

_____

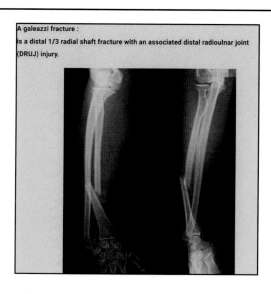

A galeazzi fracture :
is a distal 1/3 radial shaft fracture with an associated distal radioulnar joint (DRUJ) injury.

Cubital Tunnel Syndrome: Ulnar nerve compression at medial epicondyle

Sx: Pain, possible decreased grip strength

PE:

Dx: Tinel's

_____

_____

_____

Tx:

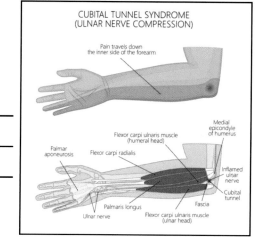

CUBITAL TUNNEL SYNDROME
(ULNAR NERVE COMPRESSION)

Pain travels down
the inner side of the forearm

Medial epicondyle of humerus

Flexor carpi ulnaris muscle (humeral head)

Flexor carpi radialis

Palmar aponeurosis

Inflamed ulnar nerve

Cubital tunnel

Fascia

Palmaris longus

Ulnar nerve

Flexor carpi ulnaris muscle (ulnar head)

Disorders of the Wrist & Hand

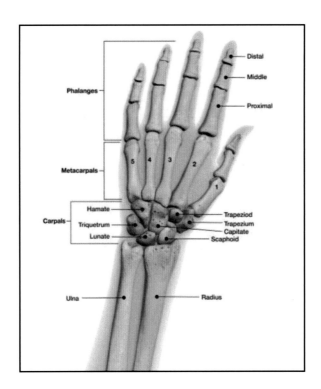

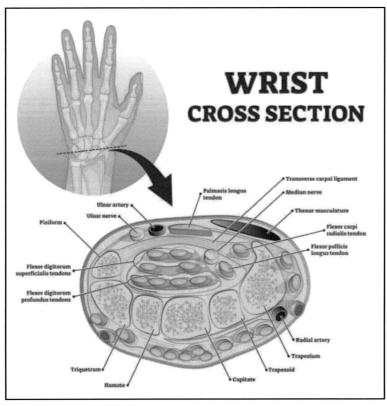

Scaphoid Fracture: **FOOSH**

Sx: Snuffbox tenderness, risk of avascular necrosis

PE:

Dx: X-ray = may not show up   MRI = definitive

    Repeat X-ray

_____   Tx:

_____

_____

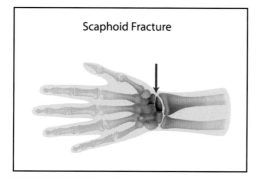

Scaphoid Fracture

Boxer Fracture:

Sx: 5th metacarpal fracture, often punching injury

PE: Check for scissoring of fingers

Dx:

_____   Tx:

_____

_____

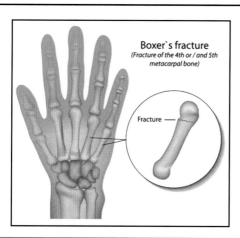

Boxer`s fracture
(Fracture of the 4th or / and 5th metacarpal bone)

Fracture

Bennett Fracture: **Usually due to axial force**

Sx: Partial fracture of 1st metacarpal

PE:

Dx: X-ray (oblique view)

Tx:

_____

_____

_____

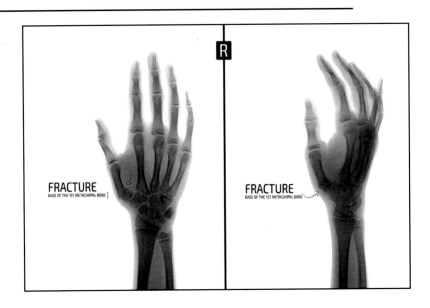

Rolando Fracture: **Prognosis worse than Bennett fracture**

Sx: Complete fracture of the 1st metacarpal, comminuted, intra-articular

PE:

Dx: X-ray (oblique view)

Tx:

_____

_____

_____

DeQuervain's Tenosynovitis: **Often from repetitive use**

Sx: Inflammation of tendon sheath at thumb MCP

PE:

Dx: Finkelstein

_____   Tx:

_____

_____

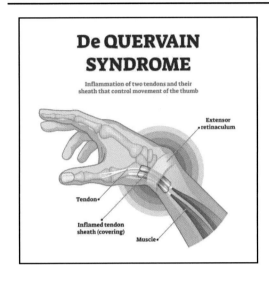

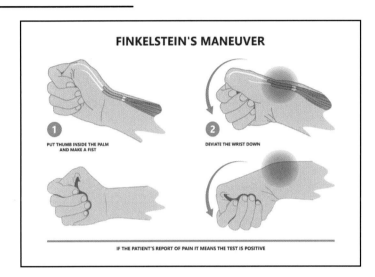

Gamekeeper's Thumb (Skier's): **Ulnar collateral ligament injury, ulnar aspect of thumb**

Sx: Pain with abduction, laxity with valgus stress, local swelling & bruising

PE:

Dx: X-ray or MRI

_____   Tx:

_____

_____

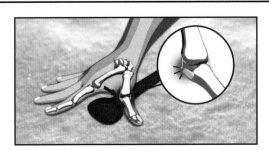

Carpal Tunnel Syndrome: Compression of median nerve at wrist, overuse injury, pregnancy can be a risk factor

Sx: Early = numbness, tingling   Late = thenar wasting

PE:

Dx: (+) Tinel, (+) Phalen

_____   Tx:

_____

_____

The Carpal Tunnel

Transverse carpal ligament

Carpal tunnel

Median nerve

Flexor tendons

Carpal bones

Colles' Fracture: Distal radius fracture, dorsal displacement of distal radius fragment, FOOSH (Outward)

Smith's Fracture: Distal radius fracture, palmar displacement of distal radius fragment, FOOSH (Inward)

Sx:

PE:

Dx: X-ray, assess for deformity and neurovascular compromise

_____   Tx:

_____

_____

Mallet Finger: Jam injury leading to flexed DIP

Sx: Joint tenderness, swelling

PE: Cannot extend DIP

Dx:

_____   Tx:

_____

_____

Boutonniere Deformity:

Sx: Joint pain, swelling, co-occurring with rheumatoid arthritis

PE: PIP flexed, DIP extended

Dx:

_____   Tx:

_____

_____

Swan Neck Deformity:

Sx: Seen in advanced RA

PE: DIP hyperflexion with PIP hyperextension

Dx:

_____   Tx:

_____

_____

Trigger Finger: **Flexor tendon locked in flexed position due to inflammation and thickening**

Sx: Cannot fully extend finger, usually episodic, usually at MCP joint

PE:

Dx:

_____   **Tx:**

_____

_____

Dupuytren's Contracture: **Fibrosis of connective tissue leading to flexed PIP**

Sx: Palmar skin changes with nodule, peritendinous cords

PE: PIP joint contracture

Dx:

_____   **Tx:**

_____

_____

Dupuytren 'S Contracture
arthritis

easy stage of the disease | the average stage of the disease | severe stage of the disease fingers not unbend

Felon: **Abscess to distal finger**

Sx: Acute infection of pulp space in fingertip, pain, fluctuant area and edema

PE:

Dx:

_____   **Tx:**

_____

_____

Paronychia:

Sx: Pain, swelling, drainage

PE:

Dx:

_____

_____

_____

Tx:

Finger Fractures:

Sx: Pain, swelling, bruising

PE:

Dx: X-ray

_____   Tx:

_____

_____

Flexor Tenosynovitis:

Sx:

PE: Kanavel's sign

Dx:

_____

_____

_____

Tx:

Kanavel's sign

Disorders of the Shoulder

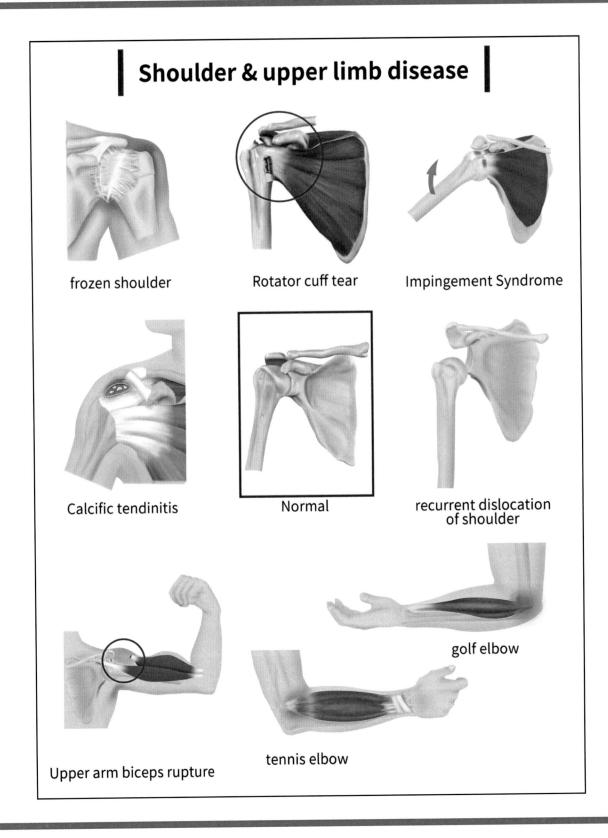

Shoulder & upper limb disease

frozen shoulder

Rotator cuff tear

Impingement Syndrome

Calcific tendinitis

Normal

recurrent dislocation of shoulder

Upper arm biceps rupture

tennis elbow

golf elbow

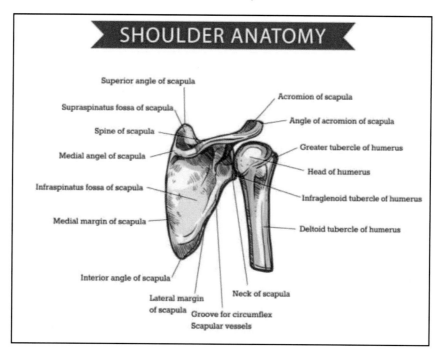

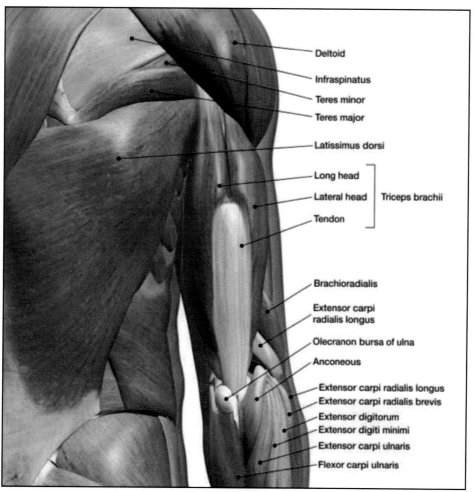

Shoulder Fracture: **Most common elderly**

Sx: Pain

PE:

Dx: X-ray

_____   Tx:

_____

_____

Bankart Lesion: **When glenoid labrum is disrupted with dislocation *associated with SLAP lesion**

Sx: Pain

PE:

Dx: X-ray

_____   Tx:

_____

_____

Hill-Sachs Lesion: **Cortical depression of humoral head made by glenoid rim**

*seen in 35-40% of anterior shoulder dislocations

Sx: Pain

PE:

Dx: X-ray

_____   Tx:

_____

_____

Shoulder Dislocation: **Most commonly anterior**

Sx: Abducted, externally rotated arm - (possible axillary nerve injury)

PE:

Dx: X-ray

_____   **Tx:**

_____

_____

Clavicle Fracture:

Sx: Swelling, pain with movement

PE:

Dx: AP X-ray

_____   **Tx:**

_____

_____

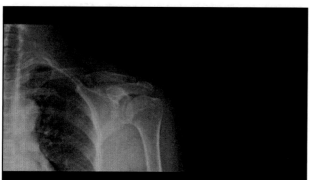

Acromioclavicular Joint Injury: **Seen after fall on shoulder**

Sx: Pain, swelling, bruising

PE:

Dx: AP X-ray

_____   Tx:

_____

_____

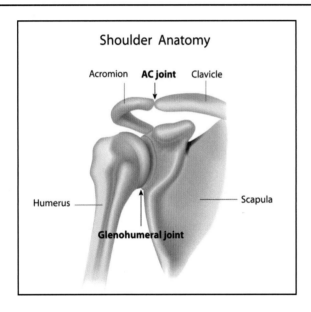

Shoulder Anatomy

Acromion   **AC joint**   Clavicle

Humerus

Glenohumeral joint

Scapula

SLAP Lesion: **Labrum tear at bicep tendon attachment (anterior to posterior)**

Sx: Clicking, catching

PE:

Dx: O'Brien test

_____   Tx:

_____

_____

Rotator Cuff Tendinopathy

Supraspinatus Tear:

Sx: Pain, weakness, diminished range of motion

PX:

Dx: (+) empty can, (+) arm drop

_____

_____   Tx:

_____

Impingement Syndrome:

Sx: Pain, weakness, diminished range of motion

PE:

Dx: (+) Hawkin's, (+) Neer's

_____   Tx:

_____

_____

Thoracic Outlet Syndrome: Compression of brachial plexus or subclavian vessels

Sx: Pain in upper extremity, paresthesia's in lower extremities

PE:

Dx: (+) Adson's test, MRI, X-ray

_____   Tx:

_____

_____

Subscapularis Tear: **Supraspinatus, infraspinatus, teres minor, subscapularis**

Sx: Pain, weakness, diminished range of motion

PE:

Dx: (+) lift off test

_____

_____

_____

Tx:

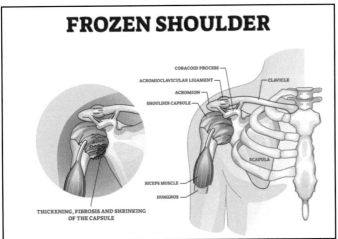

Frozen Shoulder/Adhesive Capsulitis: **Inflammation/thickening - (common with diabetes)**

Sx: Decreased ROM (active & passive)

PE:

Dx: (+) Apley scratch

_____   Tx:

_____

_____

Disorders of the Knee

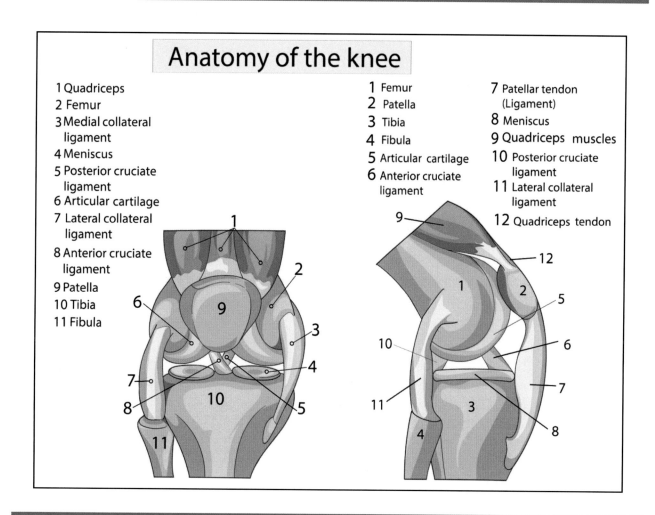

Anatomy of the knee

1 Quadriceps
2 Femur
3 Medial collateral ligament
4 Meniscus
5 Posterior cruciate ligament
6 Articular cartilage
7 Lateral collateral ligament
8 Anterior cruciate ligament
9 Patella
10 Tibia
11 Fibula

1 Femur
2 Patella
3 Tibia
4 Fibula
5 Articular cartilage
6 Anterior cruciate ligament
7 Patellar tendon (Ligament)
8 Meniscus
9 Quadriceps muscles
10 Posterior cruciate ligament
11 Lateral collateral ligament
12 Quadriceps tendon

Patellofemoral Pain Syndrome: Softening of cartilage under patella with overuse

Risk Factors: Runners or cyclists, women

Sx: Anterior knee pain behind or around the patella worsened with knee hyperflexion

PE:

Dx: (+) Patellar grind, crepitus, positive apprehension sign

_____   Tx:

_____

_____

Ligament Injuries

Anterior Cruciate Ligament (ACL): Most common pivoting injury, football & skiers

Sx: "Pop", swelling & hemarthrosis, knee buckling, inability to bear weight

PE: (+) Lachmans (more specific than anterior drawer), pivot shift test

Dx: X-ray:

    MRI:

_____   Tx:

_____

_____

Posterior Cruciate Ligament (PCL): Often with motor vehicle accidents

Sx: Posterior knee pain, anterior bruising, large effusion

PE: (+) Posterior drawer

Dx:

_____   Tx:

_____

_____

Medial Collateral Ligament (MCL) & Lateral Collateral Ligament (LCL):

Sx: Localized knee swelling, ecchymosis, stiffness

PE: MCL: Pain & laxity with (+) valgus stress

    LCL: Pain & laxity with (+) varus stress

Dx:

_____   Tx:

_____

_____

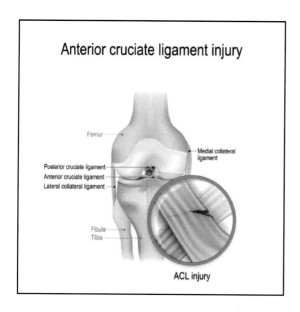

Anterior cruciate ligament injury

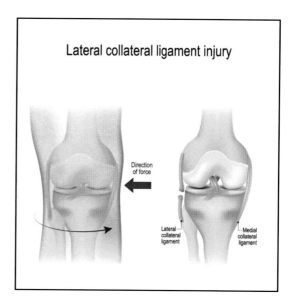

Lateral collateral ligament injury

Meniscus Tear: **Twist injury - axial loading**

Sx: Popping & giving way, swelling after activities, joint effusion

PE: (+) McMurray's, (+) Apley compression

Dx:

_____   **Tx:**

_____

_____

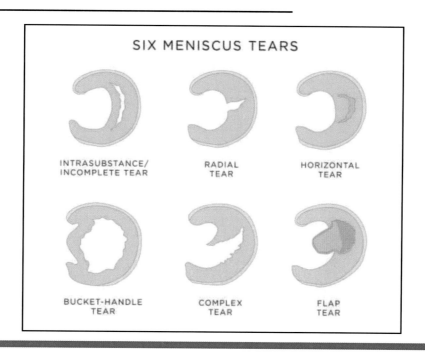

SIX MENISCUS TEARS

INTRASUBSTANCE/
INCOMPLETE TEAR   RADIAL
TEAR   HORIZONTAL
TEAR

BUCKET-HANDLE
TEAR   COMPLEX
TEAR   FLAP
TEAR

Patellar Tendonitis: **Activity related anterior knee pain, "jumper's knee"**

Sx: Tenderness inferior border of patella

PE: (+) Basset sign

Dx:

_____

_____

_____

Tx:

JUMPERS KNEE

Patellar/Quad Tendon Rupture: **Fall on flexed knee**

Sx: Inability to extend knee, sharp knee pain with ambulation

    Quadriceps:

    Patellar:

PE:

Dx: X-ray (lateral view)

    Quadriceps:

    Patellar:

_____   Tx:

_____

_____

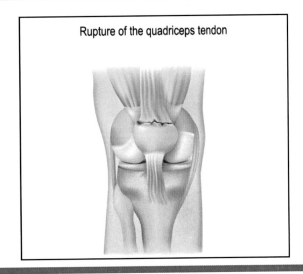

Rupture of the quadriceps tendon

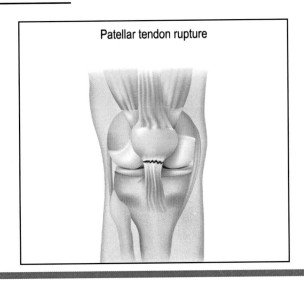

Patellar tendon rupture

Patella Dislocation: **Valgus stress after twisting injury - more common in women**

Sx: Patella displaces laterally

PE:

Dx: X-ray

_____

_____   Tx:

_____

Patella Fracture: **Usually from direct blow**

Sx: Pain, swelling, deformity, limited knee extension with pain

PE:

Dx: X-ray = sunrise view

_____

_____   Tx:

_____

Baker's Cyst: **Posterior knee cyst that contains synovial fluid**

Sx: Bulge, knee pain, swelling

PE:

Dx: Doppler to rule out DVT and see fluid

_____

_____   Tx:

_____

HEALTHY KNEE JOINT
Sagittal section of the knee

BAKER'S CYST
Sagittal section of the knee

Tibial Plateau Fractures:

Sx:

PE: Knee effusion, pain

Dx: X-ray

_____   **Tx:**

_____

_____

HEALTHY BONES OF THE KNEE	TIBIAL PLATEAU SPLIT FRACTURE	TIBIAL PLATEAU COMPRESSION FRACTURE	TIBIAL PLATEAU SPLIT AND COMPRESSION FRACTURE
Femur / Patella / Fibula / Tibia			

Femoral Condyle Fractures: **Rare**

Sx:

PE:

Dx: X-ray

_____   **Tx:**

_____

_____

Disorders of the Ankle and Foot -
Splint & Ortho follow up

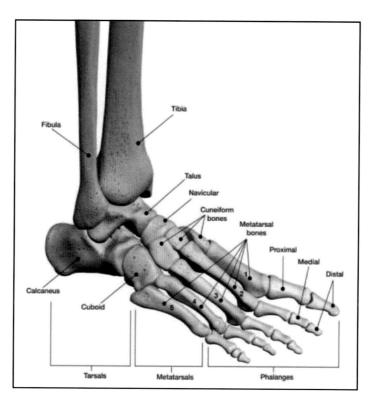

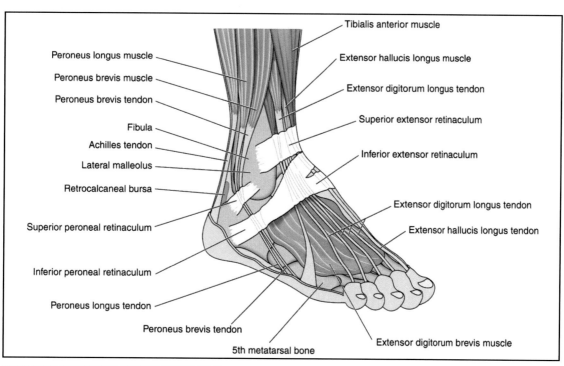

Ankle Sprain: **Most commonly the anterior talofibular ligament (ATFL)**

Sx: Grade 1:

   Grade 2:

   Grade 3:

***Always look for** Maisonneuve fracture **then** peroneal nerve involvement (foot drop and decreased sensation in digits 1 & 2)*

PE: Anterior drawer

   Talar tilt test

Dx:

_____   Tx:

_____

_____

Ankle Strain:

Sx: 1st degree: Minor tear of musculotendinous unit, swelling, local tenderness & minor loss of function

   2nd degree: More fibers torn, but without complete disruption, greater swelling & ecchymosis, loss of strength

Dx:

_____   Tx:

_____

_____

Ottawa Ankle Rule

Syndesmotic Sprain:

Sx:

PX:

Dx: X-ray

_____   Tx:

_____

_____

Achilles Tendon Rupture:

Risk Factors:

Sx: Inability to bear weight, "pop," sudden, sharp pain

PE: (+) Thompson

Dx:

_____   Tx:

_____

_____

Bunion: Hallux valgus deformity leading to lateral deviation

Risk Factors:

Sx: Pain over big toe at the MTP joint with lateral deformity

PE:

Dx:

_____

_____

_____

Tx:

Jones Fracture: Transverse fracture through the diaphysis of the 5th metatarsal

*risk for non-union & re-fracture

Sx: Pain over the fifth metatarsal with weight bearing

PE:

Dx: X-rays

_____   **Tx:**

_____

_____

Pseudo Jones: Fracture of the proximal tuberosity of the 5th metatarsal

Sx:

PE:

Dx: X-ray

_____   **Tx:**

_____

_____

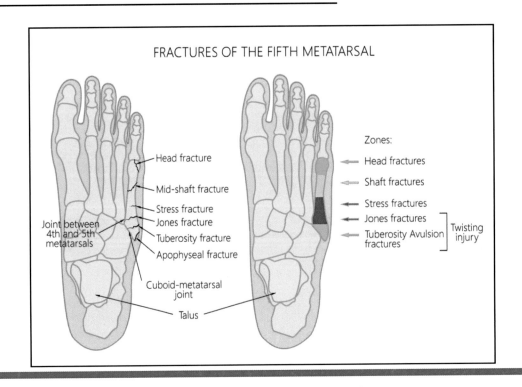

FRACTURES OF THE FIFTH METATARSAL

Head fracture

Mid-shaft fracture

Stress fracture

Jones fracture

Tuberosity fracture

Apophyseal fracture

Joint between 4th and 5th metatarsals

Cuboid-metatarsal joint

Talus

Zones:

Head fractures

Shaft fractures

Stress fractures

Jones fractures

Tuberosity Avulsion fractures

Twisting injury

Lisfranc Injury: 1+ metatarsal bone displaces from tarsus

Sx: Severe pain, inability to bear weight

PE:

Dx: X-ray - fracture at the base of the 2nd metatarsal = pathognomonic

_____   Tx:

_____

_____

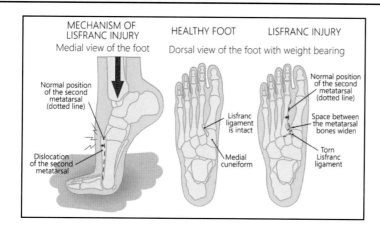

Plantar Fasciitis: Seen in athletes, one of the most common causes of foot pain in adults

Sx: Pain on plantar surface, inferior heel pain, usually worse after rest

PE: Local point tenderness, pain increases with dorsiflexion of toes

Dx:

_____   Tx:

_____

_____

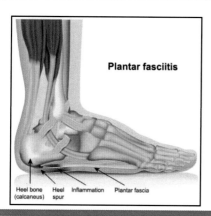

Morton's Neuroma: **Painful mass near tarsal head**

Sx: Sharp pain, possible numbness, burning pain, most common in the third intermetatarsal space

PE: Reproducible pain on palpation or squeezing the metatarsal Joints, clicking sensation "Mulder's sign"

Dx:

_____   Tx:

_____

_____

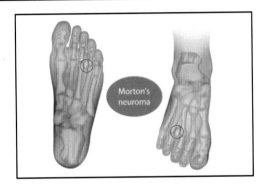

Tarsal Tunnel Syndrome: **Posterior tibial nerve compression, travels through the tarsal tunnel**

Sx: Pain increases throughout the day, worse at night, does not improve with rest

PE:

Dx:

_____   Tx:

_____

_____

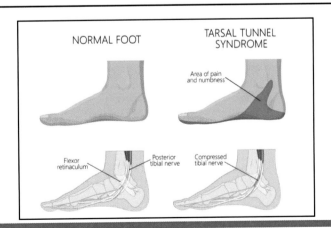

Pilon/Plafond Ankle Fracture: Distal tibia fracture from axial compression

Sx: Severe pain, swelling, deformity

PE:

Dx: X-ray

_____   Tx:

_____

_____

Maisonneuve Fracture: Fracture or rupture of the deep deltoid ligament, usually from eversion ankle injury

*Proximal fibular fracture often in conjunction with:

1. Tearing of the distal talofibular syndesmosis and the interosseous membrane

2. Medial malleolus fracture

(Anyone with a distal ankle fracture should have proximal X-ray performed to rule out Maisonneuve fracture)

Sx:

PE:

Dx: X-ray

_____   Tx:

_____

_____

Disorders of the Hip

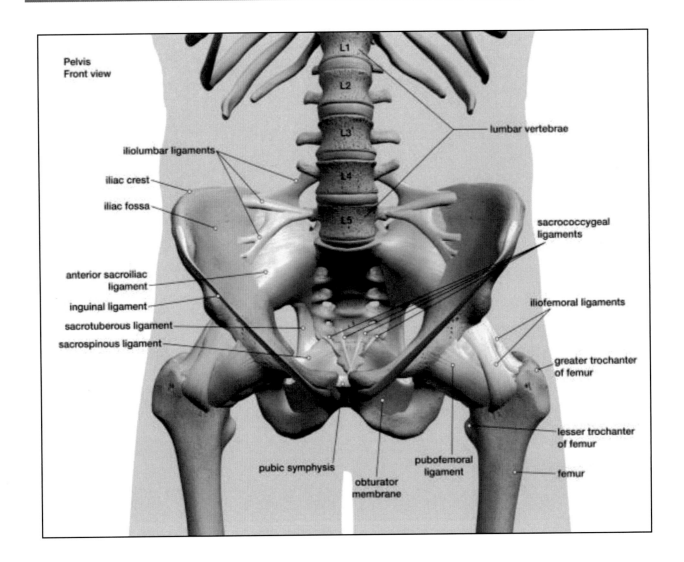

Pelvis
Front view

lumbar vertebrae

iliolumbar ligaments

iliac crest

iliac fossa

sacrococcygeal ligaments

anterior sacroiliac ligament

inguinal ligament

sacrotuberous ligament

sacrospinous ligament

iliofemoral ligaments

greater trochanter of femur

lesser trochanter of femur

pubic symphysis

pubofemoral ligament

obturator membrane

femur

Avascular Necrosis of Hip (AVN): Insidious onset hip pain

Risk Factors:

Sx:

PE:

Dx: MRI

_____   **Tx:**

_____

_____

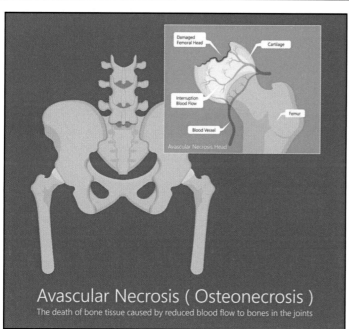

Avascular Necrosis (Osteonecrosis)
The death of bone tissue caused by reduced blood flow to bones in the joints

Legg-Calve-Perthes:

Risk Factors:

Sx: Hip pain, limp

PE:

Dx:

_____   **Tx:**

_____

_____

Hip Dislocation:

Sx: Leg shortening, internal rotation & adduction, hip pain
  Posterior:
  Anterior:

PE:

Dx: X-ray, CT

_____ **Tx:**

_____

_____

Hip Fracture: Femoral head or neck fracture, risk of avascular necrosis most common in osteoporotic women

Sx: Leg shortening, external rotation, abduction

PE:

Dx: X-ray

_____ **Tx:**

_____

_____

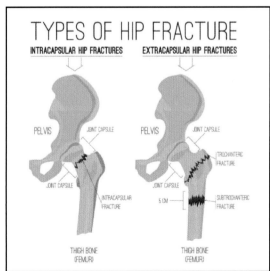

Pelvic Fractures: High impact injuries i.e., motor vehicle injuries

Sx: Pain with movement or inability to move

PE:

Dx: X-ray/CT scan

_____   Tx:

_____

_____

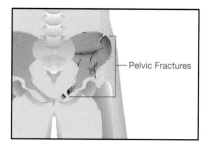

— Pelvic Fractures

Iliotibial Band Syndrome: Inflammation of the IT band

Sx: Pain over lateral femoral epicondyle

PE:

Dx: Clinical, may see signs on US

_____   Tx:

_____

_____

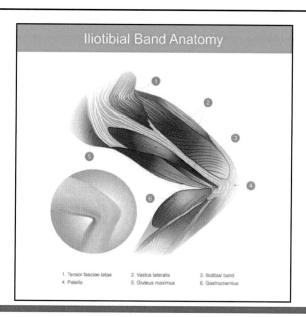

Iliotibial Band Anatomy

1. Tensor fasciae latae   2. Vastus lateralis   3. Iliotibial band
4. Patella   5. Gluteus maximus   6. Gastrocnemius

Spine Fractures

Clay Shoveler's Fracture:

Sx:

PE:

Dx: X-ray (lateral c-spine)

_____   **Tx:**

_____

_____

Hangman's Fracture:

Sx: Pain

PE:

Dx: X-ray

_____   **Tx:**

_____

_____

Jefferson Fracture: C1

Sx:

PE:

Dx: X-ray (odontoid and lateral c-spine), CT scan

_____   **Tx:**

_____

_____

Odontoid Fracture: **C2**

Sx:

PE:

Dx: X-ray (odontoid view)

_____   **Tx:**

_____

_____

Basilar Skull Fracture:

Sx: Pain

PE:

Dx: X-ray

_____   **Tx:**

_____

_____

Atlanto-Axial Joint Dislocation:

Sx:

PE:

Dx: X-ray (odontoid view) or CT

_____   **Tx:**

_____

_____

Back Disorders

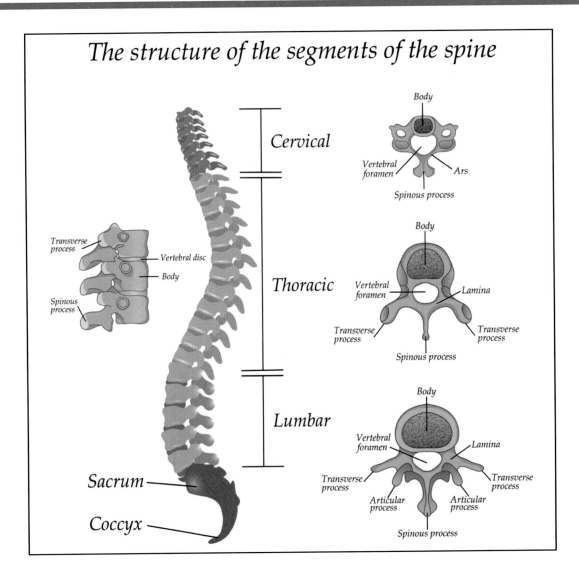

The structure of the segments of the spine

Cervical

Thoracic

Lumbar

Sacrum

Coccyx

Transverse process
Vertebral disc
Body
Spinous process

Body
Vertebral foramen
Ars
Spinous process

Body
Vertebral foramen
Lamina
Transverse process
Transverse process
Spinous process

Body
Vertebral foramen
Lamina
Transverse process
Transverse process
Articular process
Articular process
Spinous process

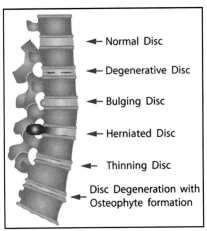

← Normal Disc

← Degenerative Disc

← Bulging Disc

← Herniated Disc

← Thinning Disc

← Disc Degeneration with Osteophyte formation

Ankylosing Spondylitis: **Seronegative spondyloarthropathy**

Sx: Back pain, stiffness, uveitis

PE:

Dx: (+) HLA-B27, bamboo spine

Healthy spine   Ankylosing spondylitis

Body of vertebra

Disc

Inflammation of joints

Fusion of bones "Bamboo spine"

_____

_____

_____

Tx:

Back Pain/Strain: **Back pain without neuro symptoms (radiculopathy)**

Sx: Pain

PE: (+) Palpation, (-) neuro exam, (-) straight leg raise, (-) Waddell's signs

Dx:

_____   Tx:

_____

_____

Cauda Equina Syndrome: **Compression of nerve roots**

Sx: Saddle anesthesia, bladder/bowel incontinence

PE:

Dx: MRI

Brain

Spinal cord

Spinal nerves

Dura and arachnoid mater

Medullary cone
Dural sac
Cauda equina

_____

_____

_____

Tx:

Herniated Nucleus Pulposus: Causes nerve roots compression
C-Spine:

Sx: Tx:

PE: (+) Spurling test

Dx:

Lumbosacral Spine:

Sx: Tx:

PE: (+) Straight leg raise

Dx:

_____

_____

_____

Spinal Stenosis: Narrowing leads to compression of nerve roots

Sx: "Shopping cart sign"

PE:

Dx: (+) Kemp sign - pain with extension

_____

_____

_____

Tx:

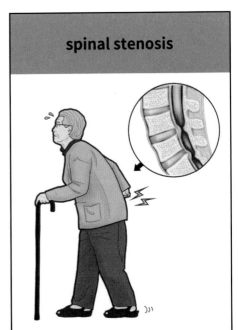
spinal stenosis

Kyphosis:

Sx:

PE: Abnormal curving of the T-spine (upper back)

Dx:

_____

_____

_____

Spondylosis: Osteoarthritis of the spine

Sx: Limitations of lumbar flexibility & tight hamstring

PE:

Dx: X-ray, MRI

_____   **Tx:**

_____

_____

Spondylolysis: **Stress fracture through pars interarticularis defect**

Sx: Limitations of lumbar flexibility & tight hamstring

PE:

Dx: X-ray, MRI

_____   Tx:

_____

_____

Spondylolisthesis: **Slipping of vertebrae (worsening of spondyloysis)**

Sx: Pain when it progresses

PE:

Dx: X-ray = "Scottie dog"

_____   Tx:

_____

_____

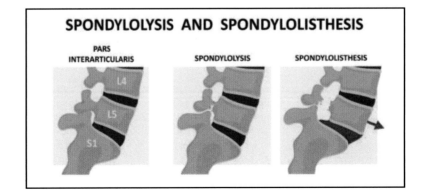

Spinal Epidural Abscess: **Most common pathogen is S. aureus**

Sx:

PE:

Dx: Spinal MRI

_____   **Tx:**

_____

_____

Epidural space (containing fat)
Vertebra
Blood vessels (venous plexus)
Spinal cord
Epidural space (containing fat)
Abscess in epidural space

Scoliosis:

Sx:

PE: Adams forward bend test, scoliometer

Dx: X-ray

_____   **Tx:**

_____

_____

Other MSK Disorders

Compartment Syndrome: Muscle & nerve ischemia

Sx:

PE: **6Ps - pain, pallor, pulselessness, paralysis, pokilothermia, paresthesia's**

Dx: Pressure > 30-45 mmHg

Tx:

_____

_____

_____

Osteoarthritis: Wear and tear

Sx: Morning stiffness, stiffness worse with use, better with rest

PE: Bouchard (PIP) vs Heberden nodes (DIP)

Dx: X-ray:

Tx:

_____

_____

_____

STAGE OF KNEE OSTEOARTHRITIS

| 10% cartilage loss | Joint-space narrowing Occurrence of osteophytes | Joint-space reduction Gaps in the cartilage | 60% of the cartilage is already lost Large osteophytes |

| I Doubtful | II Mild | III Moderate | IV Severe |

Osteoporosis: **Thinning of bony trabeculae**

Risk Factors:

Sx:

PE:

Dx: DEXA with BMD < -2.5

_____   Tx:

_____

_____

Ganglion Cyst:

Sx: Tender or non-tender dorsal wrist mass

PE:

Dx: Transillumination

_____   Tx:

_____

_____

Rhabdomyolysis: **Breakdown & necrosis of skeletal muscle**

Risk Factors:

Sx: Muscle pain & weakness, tea colored urine

PE:

Dx: CK, urinalysis, CBC, CMP, ECG

_____   **Tx:**

_____

_____

Paget's Disease: **Of bone**

Sx: Asymptomatic, bone deformity, pathologic fracture, arthritis, pain

PE:

Dx:

_____

_____

_____

Pectus Excavatum:

Sx: Sternal depression

PE:

Dx: Clinical, can do CT if severe

_____

_____

_____

Pectus Carinatum:

Sx: Protrusion of sternum

PE:

Dx: Clinical, X-ray

_____

_____

_____

Bone Tumors

Osteosarcoma: Malignant bone tumor seen in kids and adults > 65
Rare form of cancer
Most common form of cancer in patients < 20 years of age

Sx: Pain worse at night, localized bone pain

PE:

Dx: X-ray: "sunburst", "hair on ends", Codman's Triangle
  Biopsy:

Tx:

Osteosarcoma

_____

_____

_____

Ewing Sarcoma: Malignant bone tumor, most common in femur and pelvis of kids

Sx: Fever, bone pain, possibly systemic systems

PE:

Dx: X-ray: "onion skin" and/or "moth-eaten" appearance, Codman's Triangle
  Labs:

Tx:

_____

_____

_____

Chondrosarcoma: Primary malignant cartilage cancer

Sx: Constant, deep, achy pain especially @ night, _not relieved by rest_

PE:

Dx: X-ray:
  CT or MRI:

Chondrosarcoma

_____

_____

_____

Tx:

Osteochondroma: **Benign bone tumor, most common in male kids 10-20 years old**

Sx:

PE:

Dx: X-ray: pedunculated lesion in the medullary cavity

    Biopsy:

_____

_____

_____

Tx:

Fibrosarcoma: **Lytic lesions**

Sx: Painless/tender mass, pain

PE:

Dx: X-ray, MRI, CT, biopsy

_____   Tx:

_____

_____

Osteoid Osteoma: **Benign tumor in children 5-20 years old**

Sx: Increased pain @ night unrelated to activity, relieved by aspirin

PE:

Dx: X-ray: small radiolucent nidus (produces high levels prostaglandins)

    CT/MRI:

_____

_____

_____

Tx:

Infectious MSK Disorders

Osteomyelitis: Infection of the bone & marrow
Most common in femur & tibia = children
Most common in vertebrae = adults

Sx: Fever, chills, bone pain, decreased range of motion, difficulty bearing weight

PE:

Dx: Labs: increased CRP & ESR, possibly WBC

    X-ray:

    MRI:

    Bone aspiration:

_____

_____

_____

Tx:

Septic Arthritis: Bacteria in the joint cavity

Medical emergency - can rapidly destroy joints
    Knee:
    Hip:
    Sternoclavicular joint:

Sx: Swollen, warm, painful and tender joint

PE:

Dx:

    Labs:

    Arthrocentesis with WBC > 25,000:

    MRI/CT:

_____

_____

_____

Synovial Fluid Analysis:

Tx:

Rheumatologic MSK Disorders

Fibromyalgia: Widespread muscular pain

Sx: Chronic, extreme fatigue, "fibro fog", neuro symptoms, headache

PE:

Dx: Clinical diagnosis of exclusion, need 11 of 18 trigger points, normal labs

_____

_____

_____

Tx:

Sjögren's Syndrome: Autoimmune vs exocrine glands (salivary & lacrimal glands)

Sx: Dry mouth, dry eyes, vaginal dryness, bilateral parotid gland enlargement, dental caries

PE:

Dx: (+) Anti-Ro (SSA), (+) Anti-La (SSB), (+) RF, Schirmer's test < 5mm

_____

_____

_____

Tx:

Systemic Lupus Erythematosus (SLE): Multi-organ autoimmune disorder of connective tissue

Sx: Malar rash, joint pain, renal, fever, pulmonary, night sweats

    Systemic:

    Discoid Lupus:

PE:

Dx: (+) ANA, (+) anti-dsDNA & (+) anti-smith (pathognomonic & specific for SLE), antiphospholipid antibodies

_____

_____

_____

Tx:

Drug Induced Lupus:

Antiphospholipid Syndrome:

Sx: Recurrent DVT's or pulmonary embolisms, livedo reticularis

    Recurrent miscarriages, valvular heart disease, neuro symptoms (stroke, TIA)

PE:

Dx: Labs: anticardiolipin antibodies, lupus anticoagulant (increased PTT)

_____

_____

_____

Tx:

Scleroderma: Autoimmune connective tissue disorder - EXCESS Collagen

Sx: Shiny, thickened skin & tightness, interstitial lung disease, hypertension, esophageal hypomotility

    CREST:

PE:

Dx: (+) ANA, (+) anti-centromere ab, (+) anti-SCL-70 ab

_____

_____

_____

Tx: Specific to organ

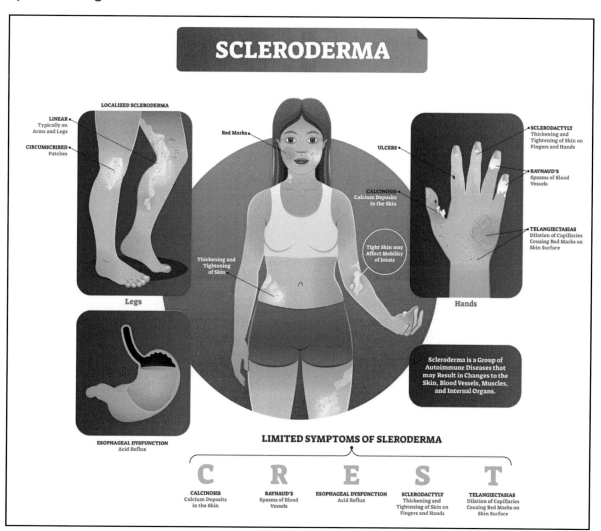

Polyarteritis Nodosa: **Small & medium vessel vasculitis of many organs**

Sx: Joint & muscle pain, Rosary sign

PE: Livedo reticularis & palpable purpura

Dx:

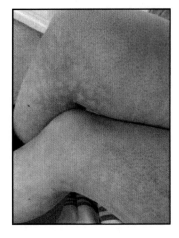

_____

_____

_____

Tx:

Rheumatoid Arthritis: **Autoimmune inflammatory disorder with symmetric polyarthritis**

Sx:

PE: Morning stiffness > 1 hour - improves later in the day
    Inflamed, small joints including MCP, PIP, MTP

Dx: Labs:
    X-ray:

_____   Tx:

_____

_____

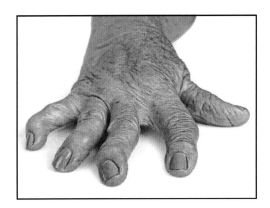

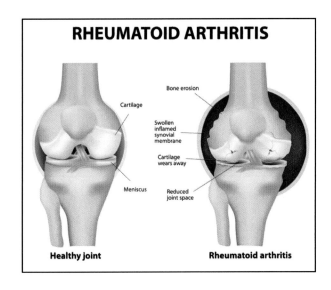

RHEUMATOID ARTHRITIS

Cartilage

Bone erosion

Swollen inflamed synovial membrane

Cartilage wears away

Meniscus

Reduced joint space

Healthy joint

Rheumatoid arthritis

Polymyositis: Idiopathic autoimmune disorder leads to inflammatory muscle disease

Sx: Progressive symmetric proximal muscle weakness (shoulders, hips)

PE:

Dx: Labs:

Muscle or skin biopsy:

_____

_____

_____

Tx:

Dermatomyositis: Polymyositis + skin involvement

Sx:

PE:

Dx: Labs:

Muscle Biopsy:

_____

_____

_____

Tx:

Dermatomyositis

Polymyalgia Rheumatica (PRM): **Inflammatory joint disease, idiopathic**

Sx: Painful synovitis, bursitis, tenosynovitis, proximal joints, worse in AM - better with movement, *associated with Giant Cell Arteritis*

PE:

Dx:

_____   Tx:

_____

_____

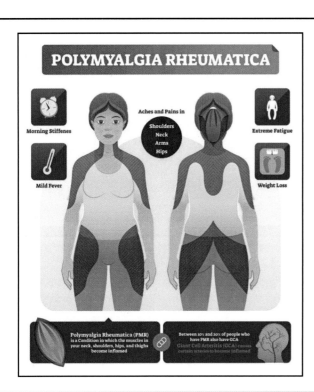

Reactive Arteritis (Reiter's): **Autoimmune response to another infection most commonly after chlamydia or shigella**

Sx: Can't see, pee or climb tree -- conjunctivitis, uveitis, urethritis, arthritis - **ASYMMETRIC**

PE:

Dx: +HLA-B27

_____   Tx:

_____

_____

Juvenile Idiopathic Arthritis: **Rheumatoid arthritis prior to age 16**
Still's disease:

Sx: Fevers, body aches, rash, hepatosplenomegaly

PE:

Dx: Labs:

_____   **Tx:**

_____

_____

Psoriatic Arthritis: **Seronegative spondylarthritis**

Sx: Dactylitis, swollen fingers, silver scaly lesions

PE:

Dx: Labs:

   X-ray:

_____   **Tx:**

_____

_____

SERONEGATIVE SPONDYLOARTHRITIS = **REACTIVE ARTERITIS, PSORIATIC ARTHRITIS, IBD, ANKYLOSING SPONDYLITIS**

Other Rheumatologic Conditions

Gout: Monosodium urate crystals

Risk Factors:

Sx: Rapid onset severe pain, joint stiffness, tenderness, tophi

PE:

Dx: Needle-shaped crystals + negative birefringence

Tx:

_____

_____

_____

Pseudogout: Calcium pyrophosphate dihydrate

Sx: Painful, tender joint

PE:

Dx:

Tx:

_____

_____

_____

Takayasu Arteritis: Large-vessel vasculitis

Sx: Syncope, chest pain, asymmetric BP in arms

PE:

Dx: Angiography with stenosis, bruit of aorta

Tx:

_____

_____

_____

Kawasaki Syndrome: Vasculitis seen in young children

Sx: CRASH and burn (conjunctivitis, rash, adenopathy, strawberry tongue, hand-foot edema, fever > 3 days)

PE:

Dx: ECHO w/ coronary artery aneurysms, high ESR & CRP

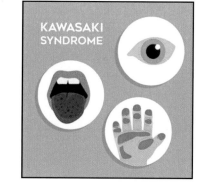

_____

_____

_____

Tx:

Granulomatosis W/Polyangiitis (Wegener's): Vasculitis

Sx: Saddle nose, chronic rhinitis, glomerulonephritis, uveitis, hoarse voice

PE:

Dx: cANCA, biopsy with granulomas

_____   Tx:

_____

_____

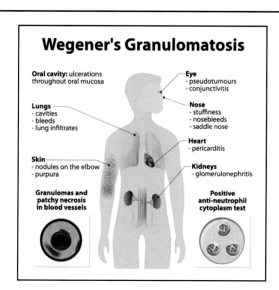

Eosinophilic Granulomatosis W/Polyangiitis (Churg-Strauss): **Small & med vessel vasculitis, lung & renal involvement**

Sx: Chronic sinusitis, asthma, blood eosinophilia

PE:

Dx: pANCA, high IgE, biopsy, ECG, ECHO

_____   Tx:

_____

_____

Microscopic Polyangiitis: **Small vessel vasculitis**

Sx: Hypertension, nephritis, pulmonary hemorrhage, purpura (no nasopharynx symptoms)

PE:

Dx: Biopsy without granulomas, increased pANCA

_____   Tx:

_____

_____

IgA Vasculitis (Henoch-Schönlein Purpura): **Small vessel vasculitis (seen in young children after URI)**

Sx: Purpura of lower extremities, nephritis

PE:

Dx: High IgA, no ANCA

_____

_____

_____

Tx:

Rheumatologic Labs

Anti-Cyclic Citrullinated Peptide: **RA**

RF: **RA**

Anti-dsDNA: **SLE**

Anti-GBM: **Goodpasture's**

Anti-Endomysial: **Celiac**

Anti-Histone: **Drug-induced SLE**

Anti-Smith: **SLE**

Anti-Jo: **Polymyositis, dermatomyositis**

Anti-Mi2: **Dermatomyositis**

Anti-Ro (SSA): **Sjögren's**

Anti-La (SSB): **Sjögren's**

Anti-SCL - 70: **Scleroderma (diffuse)**

Anti-Centromere: **CREST**

Anti-TPO: **Hashimotos**

Anti-TSI: **Grave's**

Anti-Mitochondrial: **Primary biliary cirrhosis**

pANCA: **Churg-Strauss, IBD, microscopic polyangiitis**

cANCA: **Wegener's**

HLA-B27:**(PAIR)psoriatic arthritis, ankylosing spondy, IBD, reactive arthritis**

Medications

_____: MOA = _____

Indication(s)=_____

Side Effects = _____

Types/ Examples = _____

_____

_____

_____: MOA = _____

Indication(s)=_____

Side Effects = _____

Types/ Examples = _____

_____

_____

_____: MOA = _____

Indication(s)=_____

Side Effects = _____

Types/ Examples = _____

_____

_____

_____: MOA = _____

Indication(s)=_____

Side Effects = _____

Types/ Examples = _____

_____

_____

_____: MOA = _____

Indication(s)=_____

Side Effects = _____

Types/ Examples = _____

_____

Medications

_____: MOA = _____

Indication(s)=_____

Side Effects = _____

Types/ Examples = _____

_____

_____

_____: MOA = _____

Indication(s)=_____

Side Effects = _____

Types/ Examples = _____

_____

_____

_____: MOA = _____

Indication(s)=_____

Side Effects = _____

Types/ Examples = _____

_____

_____

_____: MOA = _____

Indication(s)=_____

Side Effects = _____

Types/ Examples = _____

_____

_____

_____: MOA = _____

Indication(s)=_____

Side Effects = _____

Types/ Examples = _____

_____

EENT
Eye Disorders
All physical exams should include vision testing

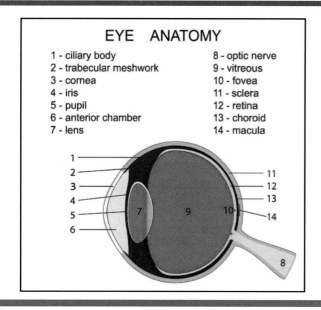

EYE ANATOMY

1 - ciliary body
2 - trabecular meshwork
3 - cornea
4 - iris
5 - pupil
6 - anterior chamber
7 - lens
8 - optic nerve
9 - vitreous
10 - fovea
11 - sclera
12 - retina
13 - choroid
14 - macula

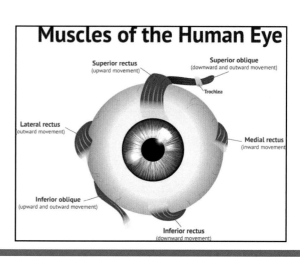

Blepharitis: Inflammation of the eyelid margin
Most common organism is S. aureus

Sx: Itching, burning, crusting of eye lids

PE:

Dx:

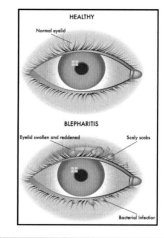

_____

_____

_____

Tx:

Blowout Fracture: Trauma related

Sx:

PE: Be sure to assess for possible inferior rectus entrapment!

Dx: CT with teardrop

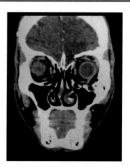

_____   Tx:

_____

_____

Cataract: **Painless opacification of lens (usually due to aging)**

Sx: Blurred cloudy vision, decreased visual acuity

PE: Absent red reflex

Dx:

_____   Tx:

_____

_____

Chalazion: **Obstruction of meibomian sebaceous gland (can be chronic)**

Sx: PAINLESS, lid swelling, slow growing

PE:

Dx:

_____   Tx:

_____

_____

Hordeolum (Stye): **Most common organism is S. aureus**

Sx: PAINFUL, edema, pustule at eyelid margin, palpable tender nodule

PE:

Dx:

_____   Tx:

_____

_____

Stye (Hordeolum)

Stye for a child   Stye at adult

Chemical Burns: **Alkali is worse than acid – *EMERGENCY!!!***

Sx:

PE:

Dx: CBC, metabolic panel, carboxyhemoglobin, arterial blood gases

Tx:

_____

_____

_____

Conjunctivitis:

Bacterial: **Most common organisms are S. aureus, S. pneumonia**

Sx: Crusting, purulent discharge

Dx:

Tx:

Viral: **Most common organism is Adenovirus**

Sx: Preauricular LAD, watery discharge

Dx:

Tx:

Allergic:

Sx: Stringy discharge, cobblestoned mucosa, bilateral erythema/irritation

Dx:

Tx:

Conjunctivitis

Corneal Abrasion:

Sx:

PE:

Dx: Fluorescein stain

_____   Tx:

_____

_____

Corneal Ulcer (Keratitis):

Bacterial Keratitis:

Sx:

PE: Hazy cornea

Dx: Limbic flush

_____   Tx:

_____

_____

HSV Keratitis:

Sx:

PE: Dendritic lesions

Dx: Conjunctival scrapings - microscope slide or culture

_____   Tx:

_____

_____

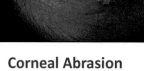
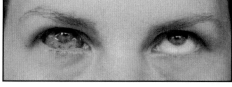
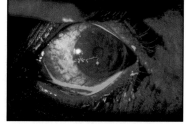

Corneal Abrasion   **Bacterial Keratitis**   **HSV Keratitis**

Ectropion: Eyelid/lashes turn outward

Most common in elderly patients

Sx: Irritation, ocular dryness, eyelid sagging

PE:

Dx:

_____   Tx:

_____

_____

Entropion: Eyelid/lashes turn inward

Most common in elderly patients

Sx: Erythema, tearing, increased sensitivity

PE:

Dx:

Entropion and Ectropion of the lower eyelid

Entropion | Healthy eye | Ectropion

_____   Tx:

_____

_____

Globe Rupture: Outer eye membranes disrupted by Trauma - EMERGENCY!!!

Sx: Enophthalmos, conjunctival hemorrhage, teardrop or irregularly shaped pupil

PE:

Dx:

_____   Tx:

_____

_____

Glaucoma: **Increased intraocular pressure, cupping, peripheral vision loss**

Acute (Angle Closure Glaucoma):

Sx: Sudden onset, painful, erythematous eye with "steamy" cornea. Fixed mid-dilated pupil, halos in vision

PE:

Dx:

_____   Tx:

_____

Chronic (Open Angle Glaucoma):

Sx: Slow onset without pain

PE:

Dx:

_____   Tx:

_____

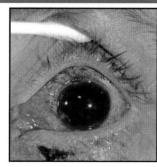

TYPES OF GLAUCOMA

OPEN-ANGLE GLAUCOMA   ANGLE-CLOSURE GLAUCOMA

Hyphema:

Sx: Blood in anterior chamber, usually due to trauma

PE:

Dx:

_____

_____

_____

Tx:

Macular Degeneration: **Most common cause of irreversible vision loss in the U.S.**

Sx: Central vision loss

PE: Dry - Drussen spots

    Wet - Neovascularization with bleeding

Dx: Amsler grid:

_____   **Tx:**

_____

_____

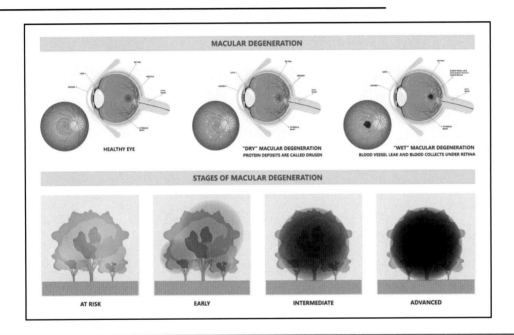

Optic Neuritis: **Associated with multiple sclerosis**

Sx: Vision loss, pain with movement, periorbital/retro-ocular pain

PE: Altered perception of color

Dx:

_____   **Tx:**

_____

_____

Orbital (Septal) Cellulitis:

Sx:

PE:

Dx: CT with contrast of sinus and orbits

_____   Tx:

_____

_____

Periorbital (Preseptal) Cellulitis: **Eyelid infection**

Sx: No pain with eye movement, eyelid erythema & edema

PE:

Dx:

NORMAL EYE

PERIORBITAL CELLULITIS

_____

_____

_____

Tx:

Papilledema: **Optic nerve swelling**
Most common cause is idiopathic

Sx:

PE:

Dx: Visual field testing, fundoscopy, MRI + LP to rule out mass

_____   Tx:

_____

_____

Pterygium:

Sx: Wing shaped conjunctival growth over cornea/pupil

PE:

Dx:

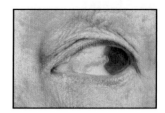

_____   **Tx:**

_____

_____

Retinal Detachment:

Sx: "Curtain drop", floaters, painless & sudden vision loss. **EMERGENCY!!!**

PE:

Dx: Fundoscopy

_____   **Tx:**

_____

_____

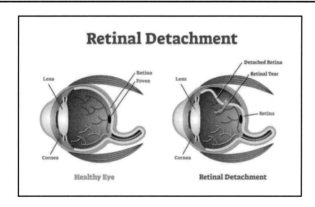

Central Retinal Artery Occlusion:

Sx: Amaurosis fugax

PE: Cherry red macula

Dx:

_____   **Tx:**

_____

_____

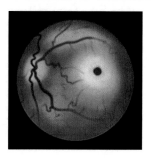

Central Retinal Vein Occlusion:

Sx: Sudden vision loss

PE:

Dx:

_____   **Tx:**

_____

_____

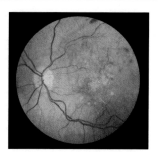

Retinopathy:

Diabetic (Non-Proliferative):

Sx: New, permanent vision loss

PE: Flame hemorrhages

Dx:

Pre-proliferative diabetic retinopathy

_____

_____

_____

Tx:

Diabetic (Proliferative): **Neovascularization**

Sx:

PE: AV nicking, cotton wool spots, concern for papilledema

Dx: Field stereoscopic fundus photography

Proliferative diabetic retinopathy

_____

_____

_____

Tx:

Hypertensive:

Sx: Vision loss

PE: Narrow arteries (copper/silver wire)

Dx:

_____

_____

_____

Tx:

Strabismus:

Sx:

PE:

Dx: Cover/uncover test

_____

_____

_____

Tx:

STRABISMUS

Hypertropia

Hypotropia

Uveitis: Inflammation of uvea

Anterior (Iritis): Most common cause is infectious

Sx: Pain, erythema, vision loss

PE:

Dx:

_____   Tx:

_____

_____

Posterior (Chorioretinitis): Most common cause is systemic inflammation

Sx:

PE:

Dx: Clinical

_____   Tx:

_____

_____

Hyperopia: "Farsighted"

Sx:

PE:

Dx:

_____   Tx:

_____

_____

Myopia: "Nearsighted"

Sx:

PE:

Dx:

_____   Tx:

_____

_____

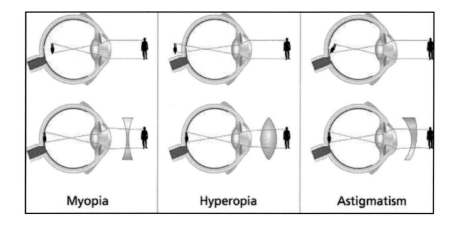

| Myopia | Hyperopia | Astigmatism |

Visual Pathways Defects

Ear Disorders

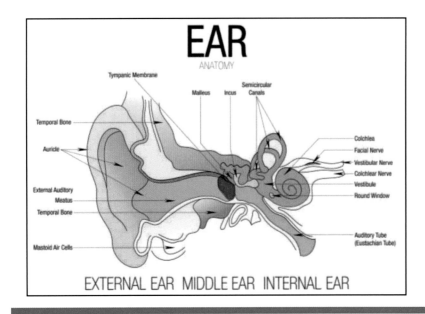

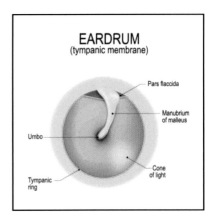

Acute Otitis Media:

Common organisms: S. pneumoniae, H. influenzae, Group A Strep

Sx:

PE: Effusion, bulging TM, decreased movement, purulent fluid behind TM, no light reflex, dull

Dx:

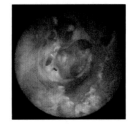

_____

_____

_____

Tx:

Chronic Otitis Media: **Tympanic membrane with perforation or otorrhea**

Sx: Otorrhea, pain, sudden "pop"

PE: Possible opening in TM

Dx:

_____

_____

_____

Tx:

Mastoiditis: Infection in mastoid air cells of the temporal bone
Most common cause: Chronic otitis media (Pseudomonas)

Sx:

PE:

Dx: CT with contrast

_____   Tx:

_____

_____

Acute Otitis Externa: "Swimmer's ear". Most common organism is Pseudomonas

Sx: Ear pain, decreased hearing

PE:

Dx: Otoscope

_____   Tx:

_____

_____

OTITIS EXTERNA

Discharge   Inflammation   Eardrum   Vestibular
            in ear canal   apparatus

Malignant Otitis Externa: Osteomyelitis at the skull base
Most common cause: Patients who are immunocomproised or have diabetes mellitus

Sx:

PE:

Dx: Otoscope visualization shows edema & erythema of ear canal
    CT/MRI/Biopsy

_____   Tx:

_____

_____

Acoustic Neuroma: **Vestibular schwannoma CN VIII**

Sx:

PE:

Dx: Audiogram, gadolinium-enhanced MRI with contrast

_____

_____

_____

Tx:

Acoustic neuroma — Vestibulocochlear nerve

Cerumen Impaction:

Sx: Diminished hearing, fullness of ear, possible otorrhea

PE:

Dx: Otoscope

_____   **Tx:**

_____

_____

Cholesteatoma: **Keratinized desquamated epithelium**

Sx:

PE:

Dx: Otoscope visualization shows granulation tissue

_____

_____

_____

Tx:

Cholesteatoma

Healthy eardrum   Eardrum is perforated and retracted   Cholesteatoma

Eustachian Tube Dysfunction: **Often found with viral URI, allergic rhinitis, or barotrauma**

Sx: Hearing loss, aural fullness, complaints of "can't pop ears"

PE:

Dx:

_____   Tx:

_____

_____

Hearing Loss

Conductive Hearing Loss: **Most common cause is cerumen impaction**

Sx:

PE:

Dx: Weber lateralizes to affected side. Rinne shows bone conduction > air conduction

_____   Tx:

_____

_____

Sensorineural Hearing Loss: **Most common cause of hearing loss in adults**

Sx:

PE:

Dx: Weber lateralizes to "good" ear. Rinne shows air conduction > bone conduction

_____   Tx:

_____

_____

Auricular Hematoma: **Usually related to trauma**

Sx: Physical deformity, swelling and/or bruising of the auricle

PE:

Dx:

_____   Tx:

_____

_____

Otosclerosis: **Abnormal bony overgrowth of stapes**

Sx: Slow, progressive conductive hearing loss and tinnitus

PE:

Dx:

_____   **Tx:**

_____

_____

Tinnitus: **Ringing in ears**

Sx:

PE:

Dx: Audiometry

_____   **Tx:**

_____

_____

Tympanic Membrane Perforation:

Sx: Otorrhea, ear pain, decreased hearing in affected ear

PE:

Dx:

_____   **Tx:**

_____

_____

Tympanosclerosis: **Scarring of the eradrum**

Sx: Small white area on TM (usually from perforation or tubes)

PE:

Dx:

_____   **Tx:**

_____

_____

Vertigo

Peripheral: Vestibular

Sx: False sense of motion (or exaggerated sense of motion)

PE:

Dx:

_____   Tx:

_____

_____

Vestibular system

Central: Brainstem & cerebellum

More common in patients with multiple sclerosis & ischemic posterior circulation stroke

Sx:

PE:

Dx: Gait issues, positive CNS signs, non-fatigable vertical nystagmus

_____   Tx:

_____

_____

Benign Paroxysmal Positional Vertigo (BPPV): Displaced otoliths (small calcium carbonate crystals on cilia)

Sx: Lasting second to minutes

PE:

Dx: + Dix-Hallpike (fatigable nystagmus)

_____   Tx:

_____

_____

Ménière's Disease: Excess endolymph in inner ear

Sx: Vertigo for minutes to hours, low frequency sensorineural hearing loss + tinnitus + pressure

PE:

Dx: Transtympanic electrocochleography, caloric testing

_____   Tx:

_____

_____

Vestibular Neuritis: **Inflammation of vestibular portion of CN VIII**
Common causes: Viral infection

Sx: Lasting days to weeks

PE:

Dx: Clinical, MRI to rule out other possible causes

_____   Tx:

_____

_____

Labyrinthitis: **Inflammation of vestibular & cochlear portion of CN VIII**

Sx: Symptoms of vestibular neuritis + unilateral hearing loss + tinnitus

PE:

Dx:

_____   Tx:

_____

_____

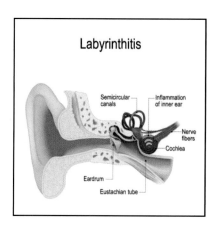

Nose/Sinus Disorders

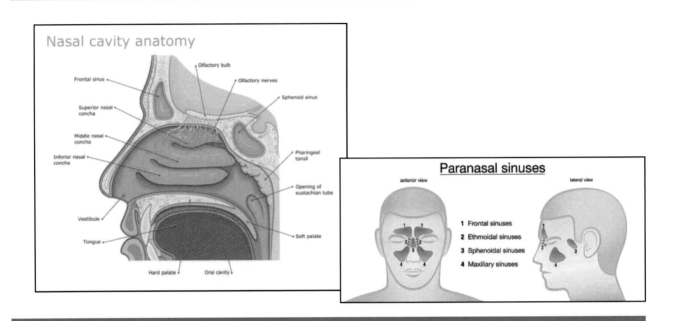

Rhinosinusitis (Acute Sinusitis): More common in maxillary sinuses

Common organisms: S. pneumoniae, H. influenzae, Group A strep

Sx: Rhinorrhea, sinus pain, referred dental pain

PE:

Dx:

_____

_____

_____

Tx:

Chronic Sinusitis: 12+ weeks of symptoms

Sx: Same as acute sinusitis

PE:

Dx: CT

_____   Tx:

_____

_____

Allergic Rhinitis: IgE

Sx:

PE: Pale, blue, boggy, nares with cobblestoning. May have nasal polyps

Dx: Trial of antihistamine or intranasal corticosteroid, allergy testing

_____ Tx:

_____

_____

Mechanism OF Allergic

Exposure to allergen | IgE prouduction, attach to mast cell | Allergen attachment, mast cell release histamines | Allergic

Foreign Body: Most common in kids

Sx: Foul smelling nares, epistaxis, mucopurulent discharge

PE:

Dx:

_____ Tx:

_____

_____

Nasal Polyps: More common in patients with allergic rhinitis
Samter's Triad: Asthma, nasal polyps, Aspirin/NSAID sensitivity/allergy

Sx:

PE:

Dx:

_____ Tx:

_____

_____

Epistaxis

Anterior: **Kiesselbach's plexus (more common with trauma)**

Sx:

PE:

Dx: Clinical

_____   Tx:

_____

_____

Posterior: **Sphenopalatine artery (posterior pharynx)**

Sx: Blood in both nares and posterior pharynx

PE:

Dx:

_____   Tx:

_____

_____

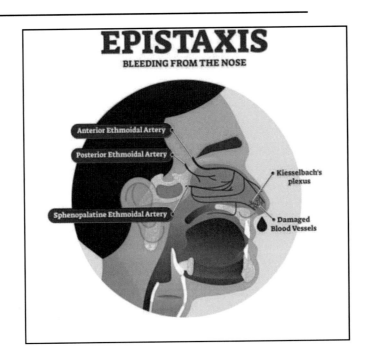

Throat Disorders

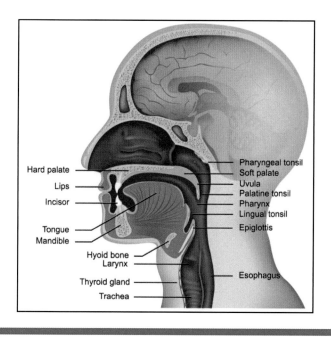

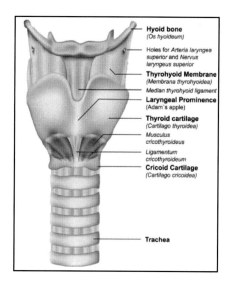

Acute Pharyngitis/Tonsillitis: **Bacterial (Group A Strep)**

Most common overall cause is viral

Complications:

Scarlet fever:

Rheumatic fever:

Sx: Scarlatina rash, exudates, no cough, sore throat, difficulty swallowing

PE:

Dx:

Tx:

_____

_____

_____

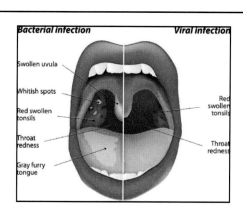

Aphthous Ulcer: "Canker sore"

Sx: Painful, shallow ulcer with yellow, white or grey central exudate and surrounding erythema

PE:

Dx:

_____   Tx:

_____

_____

Croup (Parainfluenza):

Sx: Barking cough, inspiratory stridor, hoarseness

PE:

Dx:

_____   Tx:

_____

_____

Epiglottitis: **Most common cause is H. flu**

Sx: Dysphagia, inspiratory stridor, tripod, drooling, muffled "hot potato" voice

PE:

Dx:

_____   Tx:

_____

_____

Laryngitis:

Common causes: Viral upper respiratory infection, bacterial infection, trauma

Sx: Hoarseness, aphonia, dry scratchy throat, runny nose, cough, sore throat

PE:

Dx:

_____   Tx:

_____

_____

Ludwig's Angina: Cellulitis of sublingual or submaxillary space
Most common cause: Dental infection

Sx: Swelling, "woody" induration, pus

PE:

Dx:

_____   Tx:

_____

_____

Oral Candidiasis (Thrush):

Sx:

PE:

Dx: Clinical. KOH shows budding yeast & pseudo hyphae

_____   Tx:

_____

_____

Erythroplakia: **High risk of malignant transformation**
Risk Factor: Cigarette smoking

Sx: Painless, erythematous, soft, velvety, patch in mouth

PE:

Dx:

_____   Tx:

_____

_____

Oral Leukoplakia: **Caused by Epstein-Barr virus. More common in immunocompromised patients**

Sx: Painless white plaque along lateral tongue border or buccal mucosa

PE:

Dx:

_____   Tx:

_____

_____

Oral Hairy Leukoplakia:

Sx: Painless, erythematous, soft, velvety, patch in mouth

PE:

Dx:

_____   Tx:

_____

_____

Oral Lichen Planus: **Autoimmune or Hepatits C (most common causes)**

Sx: Lacy reticular leukoplakia (Wickham striae), erythematous ulcers

PE:

Dx:

_____   Tx:

_____

_____

Peritonsillar Abscess:

Most common organisms: Group A Strep, S. aureus, polymicrobial

Sx: "Hot potato" voice, drooling, trismus, uvula to contralateral side

PE:

Dx:

_____

_____

_____

Tx:

TONSILS AND THROAT DISEASES
PERITONSILLAR ABSCESS

Retropharyngeal Abscess:

Sx: Difficulty and pain with swallowing, fever, stiff neck, drooling, difficulty breathing

PE:

Dx:

_____

_____

_____

Tx:

Parotitis/Sialadenitis: Inflammation of salivary glands
Most common infectious cause:
Most common bacterial cause:

Sx: Sudden onset, dysphagia, trismus. Tenderness, swelling, and purulent discharge of salivary glands

PE:

Dx:

_____   Tx:

_____

_____

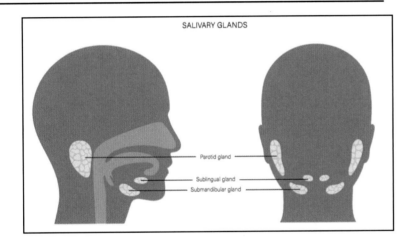

Sialolithiasis: Most common at Wharton's ducts (submandibular gland) and Stensen's duct (parotid gland)

Sx: Post prandial salivary gland pain and swelling

PE:

Dx:

_____   Tx:

_____

_____

EENT Neoplasms

Nasopharyngeal Carcinomas: **Associated with tobacco, EtOH, EBV**

Sx: Difficulty speaking, breathing, hearing

PE:

Dx:

_____   Tx:

_____

_____

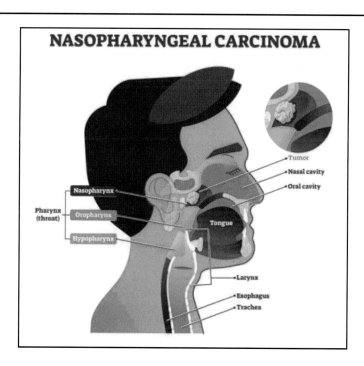

Herpes Simplex Virus 1: **In ID**

Medications

_____: MOA = _____

Indication(s)=_____

Side Effects = _____

Types/ Examples = _____

_____

_____

_____: MOA = _____

Indication(s)=_____

Side Effects = _____

Types/ Examples = _____

_____

_____

_____: MOA = _____

Indication(s)=_____

Side Effects = _____

Types/ Examples = _____

_____

_____

_____: MOA = _____

Indication(s)=_____

Side Effects = _____

Types/ Examples = _____

_____

_____

_____: MOA = _____

Indication(s)=_____

Side Effects = _____

Types/ Examples = _____

_____

Medications

_____: MOA = _____

Indication(s)=_____

Side Effects = _____

Types/ Examples = _____

_____

_____

_____: MOA = _____

Indication(s)=_____

Side Effects = _____

Types/ Examples = _____

_____

_____

_____: MOA = _____

Indication(s)=_____

Side Effects = _____

Types/ Examples = _____

_____

_____

_____: MOA = _____

Indication(s)=_____

Side Effects = _____

Types/ Examples = _____

_____

_____

_____: MOA = _____

Indication(s)=_____

Side Effects = _____

Types/ Examples = _____

_____

Infectious Disease
Viral Diseases

Herpes Simplex Virus 1: "Cold sore"

Sx: Tingling sensation (prodrome), vesicles can cross vermillion border

PE:

Dx:

_____

_____

_____

Tx:

Herpes Simplex Virus 2: Genital lesions/ulcers

Sx: Painful ulcers and/or vesicular lesions that progress to ulcerations

PE:

Dx:

_____

_____

_____

Tx:

Herpes Simplex Virus 3 (Varicella Zoster "VZV" or "Shingles"):

Sx:

PE:

Dx: Clinical, Tzanck smear, polymerase chain reaction (PCR)

_____

_____

_____

Tx:

Herpes Simplex Virus 4 (Epstein-Barr virus "EBV"): **Mononucleosis**

Complications:

Sx: Fever + posterior cervical lymphadenopathy + pharyngitis, splenomegaly

PE:

Dx:

_____   **Tx:**

_____

_____

Herpes Simplex Virus (Cytomegalovirus "CMV"): **Mononucleosis**

Sx: Malaise, fever, N/V/D

PE:

Dx:

_____   **Tx:**

_____

_____

Herpes Simplex Virus 6 & 7 (Roseola "6th disease"):

Sx: Fever, exanthem rash

PE:

Dx:

_____

_____

_____

Tx:

Herpes Simplex Virus 8 (Kaposi Sarcoma): **AIDS related**

Sx: Skin lesion (purple), oral lesion, LAD, weight loss

PE:

Dx:

_____   **Tx:**

_____

_____

Human Immunodeficiency Virus (HIV): **Retrovirus**
AIDS: CD4 < 200 w/opportunistic infection

Sx: Fever, night sweats, weight loss, skin rashes, oral ulcers

PE:

Dx: ELISA (sensitive), Western blot (specific)

_____   **Tx:**

_____

_____

Human Papillomavirus (HPV): Linked to cervical & oropharyngeal cancers
Types: Cutaneous warts (1,2,4), genital warts (6, 11), cancerous (16, 18)

Sx:

PE:

Dx: Biopsy, PAP smear

_____

_____

_____

Tx:

CERVICAL CANCER

Cervical cancer

Human papillomavirus

Mumps: Paramyxovirus

Complications: Orchitis, aseptic meningitis, pancreatitis

Sx:

PE:

Dx: Elevated amylase, leukopenia, + IgM and IgG.

_____   **Tx:**

_____

_____

Rabies: CNS infection

Transmission: Via animals including unvaccinated house pets (dogs)

Sx:

PE:

Dx: Gram stain negri bodies, polymerase chain reaction (PCR)

_____   **Tx:**

_____

_____

Parasitic Diseases

Amebiasis (Entamoeba Histolytica): **Protozoa**

Sx:

PE:

Dx: Stool antigen, serum antibody

_____   Tx:

_____

_____

Malaria: **Protozoa**

Protective Factors: Sickle cell trait and thalassemia trait

Sx: Cyclical fever (3 days), anemia, coma

PE:

Dx: Giemsa stain smear

_____   Tx:

_____

_____

Babesiosis: **Protozoa**
Transmission: Ticks

Sx: Fever, hemolytic anemia, jaundice

PE:

Dx:

_____   Tx:

_____

_____

Toxoplasmosis: Protozoa

Transmission: Cat feces & raw pork

Congenital: Blueberry muffin rash

Sx:

PE:

Dx: Anti-Toxoplasma IgG (serum) & IgM (serum)

_____   **Tx:**

_____

_____

Chagas Disease (American Trypanosomiasis): Trypanosoma cruzi (T. cruzi)

Sx: Acute-

    Latent-

PE:

Dx: CBC, microscopy

_____   **Tx:**

_____

_____

Trichinellosis: Roundworm

Transmission: Consumption of raw pork

Sx: Periorbital/facial edema, myositis, fever

PE:

Dx:

_____   **Tx:**

_____

_____

Ascariasis: Roundworm

Transmission: Poor sanitation, travel to endemic areas

Sx:

PE:

Dx: Stool microscopy, chest or abdominal X-ray

_____   **Tx:**

_____

_____

Enterobius (Pinworms):
Transmission: Fecal-oral, thumb sucking

Sx: Perianal itching (worse at night) & perianal erythema

PE:

Dx: Scotch tape test

_____   Tx:

_____

_____

Cestodes (Tapeworms):

Sx: GI symptoms, weight loss, seizures, hepatomegaly

PE:

Dx:

_____   Tx:

_____

_____

Hookworms:
Transmission: Enter through feet from infected soil, goes into lungs, gets coughed up then swallowed into gastrointestinal tract

Sx:

PE:

Dx: Clinical = skin scrapings/biopsy, eggs in feces

_____   Tx:

_____

_____

Leishmaniasis: Sandfly bite (protozoa)

Sx: Cutaneous ulcers, visceral hepatosplenomegaly, fever

PE:

Dx: CBC, LFT's, BUN, hCG

_____   Tx:

_____

_____

Fungal Diseases

Candidiasis:

Sx: Esophagitis, oral thrush, vaginal, fungemia, endocarditis

PE:

Dx: KOH with budding yeast and pseudohyphae

_____   Tx:

_____

_____

Cryptococcosis: Most common in patients with HIV infection and immunosuppression
Transmission: Pigeon droppings

Sx: Meningitis, pneumonia, constitutional symptoms

PE:

Dx:

_____   Tx:

_____

_____

Histoplasmosis: Michigan & Ohio River Valley, most common in patients with AIDS
Transmission: Bat and bird droppings

Sx: Fever, headache, non-productive cough, pleuritic chest pain

PE:

Dx:

_____   Tx:

_____

_____

Pneumocystis: P. jirovecii, most common in patients with AIDS (CD4 cell count < 200 cells/microliter)

Sx:

PE:

Dx: Chest X-ray with bilateral peri-hilar infiltrates, high LDH

_____   Tx:

_____

_____

Aspergillosis:

Sx:

PE:

Dx: Chest X-ray, high-resolution chest CT scan, MRI of brain & sinuses

_____   **Tx:**

_____

_____

Mucormycosis:

Sx: Sinus and facial pain, proptosis, skin nodules, black eschars

PE:

Dx:

_____   **Tx:**

_____

_____

Coccidioidomycosis: "Valley fever", southwestern USA

Sx:

PE:

Dx: Sputum culture, enzyme immunoassay serology

_____   **Tx:**

_____

_____

Blastomycosis: Pulmonary, cutaneous, disseminated

Sx: Fever, weight loss, fatigue, cough, skin lesion

PE:

Dx:

_____   **Tx:**

_____

_____

Bacterial Respiratory Diseases

Diphtheria: Corynebacterium diphtheria (gram-positive rod)

Sx: Sore throat, pseudo membrane formation, neck swelling

PE:

Dx:

_____   **Tx:**

_____

_____

Mycobacterium Avium Complex: Prior lung disease, most common in patients with AIDS

Sx:

PE:

Dx: CBC, LFT, sputum culture (acid fast), X-ray

_____   **Tx:**

_____

_____

Other Bacterial Diseases

Methicillin-Resistant Staphylococcus Aureus (MRSA): S. aureus resistant to methicillin (usually various other drugs) most common in immunocompromised patients or IV drug users

Sx: Skin lesions - pustules on an erythematous base, gold/salmon sputum

PE:

Dx:

_____   Tx:

_____

_____

**Rocky Mountain Spotted Fever: Rickettsia ricketsii (gram-negative, obligate intracellular)
Transmission: Ticks**

Sx: Centripetal rash (outside in), fever, rash, headache

PE:

Dx:

_____   Tx:

_____

_____

**Erythema Migrans (Lyme Disease): Borrelia burgdorferi (gram-negative spirochete)
Transmission: Deer tick**

Sx: Bull's eye rash, cardiac arrythmias, chronic arthritis
    Early disease vs. late disease

PE:

Dx:

_____

_____

_____

Tx:

Zika: **Transmitted by mosquitos**
Dangerous in pregnancy

Sx:

PE:

Dx: Reverse transcriptase-polymerase chain reaction (RT-PCR), serology

_____   **Tx:**

_____

_____

Cat Scratch: **Bartonella henselae (gram-negative coccobacillli)**

Sx: Ulcer, fever, lymphadenopathy, papular or pustular lesion

PE:

Dx: Serology, culture

_____   **Tx:**

_____

_____

Tularemia: **Gram-negative coccobacillli**
Transmission: Tick, biting fly, rabbits, and other infected animals

Sx:

PE:

Dx: Serology, blood and specimen culture, PCR of ulcer or lymph

_____   **Tx:**

_____

_____

Brucellosis: Gram-negative coccobacilli

Transmission: Infected animal products, usually milk or cheese

Sx: Fever, chills, constitutional symptoms, arthralgias

PE:

Dx:

_____ Tx:

_____

_____

Plague: Yersinia pestis (gram-negative rod)

Sx: Bubonic:

Yersiniosis:

Pneumonic:

Dx: Bubonic:

Pneumonic:

Yersiniosis:

_____ Tx:

_____

_____

Necrotizing Fasciitis:

Sx: Bullae, gangrene, fever, nausea, vomiting

PE:

Dx:

_____ Tx:

_____

_____

Bacterial STIs

Chlamydia: Obligate intracellular gram-negative rod

Sx: White discharge or asymptomatic, white cervical or penile discharge, friable cervix

PE: Post-coital bleeding (female)

Dx:

_____

Tx:

_____

_____

Gonorrhea: Neisseria gonorrhoeae (gram-negative diplococci)

Sx: Asymptomatic OR yellow, purulent discharge,
   urethritis, cervicitis, epididymitis, prostatitis,
   risk of pelvic inflammatory disease (PID) in women

PE:

Dx:

_____

Tx:

_____

_____

Syphilis: Treponema pallidum (spirochete)

Sx: 1. Primary:

   2. Secondary:

   3. Tertiary:

Congenital - Hutchinson teeth, saddle-nose deformity, keratitis

Dx: Darkfield microscopy of chancre

   Sensitive:

   Specific:

_____

Tx:

_____

_____

Chancroid: **Haemophilus ducreyi (gram-negative coccobacillus)**

Sx: Painful genital ulcers, inguinal lymphadenopathy

PE:

Dx:

_____   Tx:

_____

_____

Lymphogranuloma Venereum (LGV):

Sx: Inguinal lymphadenopathy, fever, malaise, arthralgias, lower abdominal or lower back pain

    Stage 1:

    Stage 2:

    Stage 3:

PE:

Dx: NAAT (genital or lymph node specimens)

_____   Tx:

_____

_____

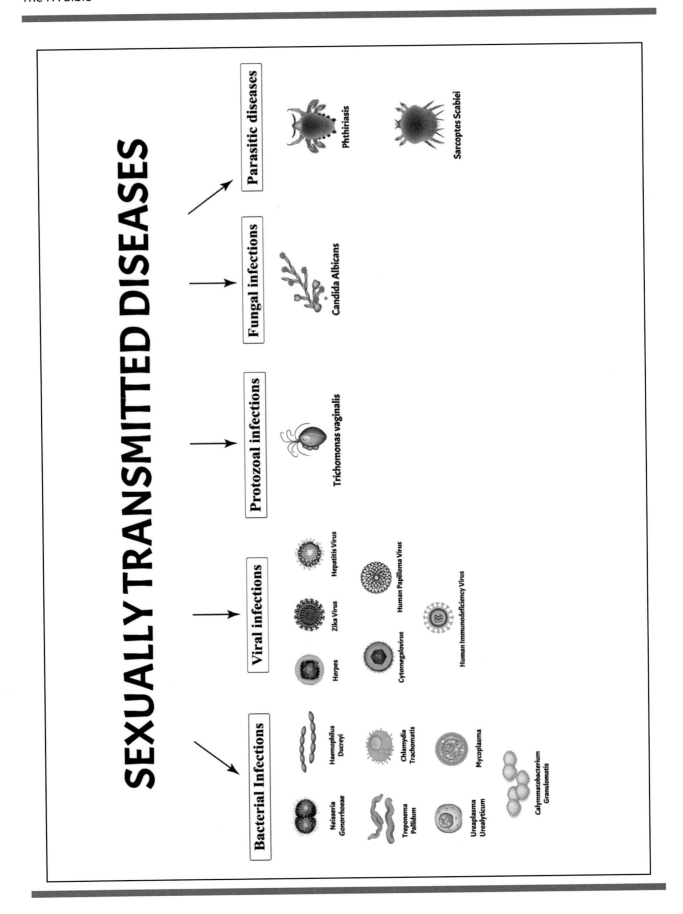

SEXUALLY TRANSMITTED DISEASES

Bacterial Infections

Neisseria Gonorrhoeae
Haemophilus Ducreyi
Treponema Pallidum
Chlamydia Trachomatis
Ureaplasma Urealyticum
Mycoplasma
Calymmatobacterium Granulomatis

Viral infections

Herpes
Zika Virus
Hepatitis Virus
Cytomegalovirus
Human Papilloma Virus
Human Immunodeficiency Virus

Protozoal infections

Trichomonas vaginalis

Fungal infections

Candida Albicans

Parasitic diseases

Phthiriasis
Sarcoptes Scabiei

Bacterial Gastrointestinal Diseases

Campylobacter Jejuni: Gram-negative curved rod

Transmission: Contaminated meat or milk

Sx: Abdominal pain, diarrhea, headache, myalgias, chills, fever

PE:

Dx:

_____   Tx:

_____

_____

Botulism: Clostridium botulinum (gram-positive, anaerobic rod with spores)

Transmission:

Sx: Flaccid paralysis, respiratory distress, "floppy baby" syndrome

PE:

Dx:

Botulinum Toxin Poisoning

Healthy Neuromuscular Junction

Neuromuscular Junction with Botulinum Poisoning

_____

_____

_____

Tx:

Anthrax: Gram-positive rod with spores

Sx:

PE:

Dx:

_____   Tx:

_____

_____

Bacterial Neurologic Diseases

Tetanus: Gram-positive, anaerobic rod, neurotoxin

Sx: Trismus (lock jaw), back pain, dysphagia, muscle spasms

PE:

Dx:

_____   Tx:

_____

_____

Meningococcal Meningitis: Neisseria meningitides (gram-negative diploccoci)

Sx: Nuchal rigidity + fever + HA, purpuric rash

    (+) Kernig's:

    (+) Brudzinski's:

PE:

Dx:

MENINGITIS
Scull
Dura mater
Inflammation
Arachnoid mater
Pia mater
Brain
Meninges
Neisseria meningitidis
Brain

_____

_____

_____

Tx:

Listeriosis: Gram-positive rod

Common causes: Exposure to contaminated food

Sx:

PE:

Dx: CBC, brain MRI & CT

_____   Tx:

_____

_____

Vaginal Infections

Candida Vaginitis:

Sx: Thick, curdy, white discharge

PE:

Dx: Wet mount = pseudo hyphae "spaghetti & meatballs"

_____   Tx:

_____

_____

Bacterial Vaginosis:

Sx: Thin, white/grey discharge

PE:

Dx: Wet mount = clue cells

_____   Tx:

_____

_____

Trichomoniasis:

Sx: Frothy, green/yellow discharge

PE:

Dx: Wet mount = motile trichomonads

_____

_____

_____

Tx:

Trichomonas

Flagella

Cytosome

Nucleus

Undulating membrane

Vacuole

Axostyle

Pelvic Inflammatory Disease (PID):

Sx:

PE: Chandelier sign (cervical motion tenderness), adnexal mass

Dx: Labs = high WBC > 10,000, fever

_____

_____

_____

Tx:

Tubo-Ovarian Abscess: **Usually follows PID**

Sx:

Dx: Pelvic US

_____   Tx:

_____

_____

---

*Mycoplasma Pneumoniae: **In Pulm***

*Pertussis "Whooping Cough": **In Pulm***

*Tuberculosis: **In Pulm***

*Rheumatic Fever: **In Cardio***

*Cholera: **In GI***

*Pharyngitis (Strep Throat): **In EENT***

*Pityriasis Rosea: **In Derm***

*Haemophilus Influenzae: **In Pulm***

*Salmonella: **In GI***

*Shigella: **In GI***

*Condyloma Acuminatum: **In Derm***

Medications

_____ : MOA = _____

Indication(s)=_____

Side Effects = _____

Types/ Examples = _____

_____

_____

_____ : MOA = _____

Indication(s)=_____

Side Effects = _____

Types/ Examples = _____

_____

_____

_____ : MOA = _____

Indication(s)=_____

Side Effects = _____

Types/ Examples = _____

_____

_____

_____ : MOA = _____

Indication(s)=_____

Side Effects = _____

Types/ Examples = _____

_____

_____

_____ : MOA = _____

Indication(s)=_____

Side Effects = _____

Types/ Examples = _____

_____

Medications

_____: MOA = _____

Indication(s)=_____

Side Effects = _____

Types/ Examples = _____

_____

_____

_____: MOA = _____

Indication(s)=_____

Side Effects = _____

Types/ Examples = _____

_____

_____

_____: MOA = _____

Indication(s)=_____

Side Effects = _____

Types/ Examples = _____

_____

_____

_____: MOA = _____

Indication(s)=_____

Side Effects = _____

Types/ Examples = _____

_____

_____

_____: MOA = _____

Indication(s)=_____

Side Effects = _____

Types/ Examples = _____

_____

Dermatology

Atopic Dermatitis (Eczema):

Sx: Asthma, allergic rhinitis, pruritis, erythema, scaling, vesicles, papules
   FLEXOR SURFACES

PE:

Dx:

_____

_____

_____

Tx:

Dyshidrotic Eczema:

Sx: Tapioca-like bumps, itchy, symmetric

PE:

Dx:

_____

_____

_____

Tx:

Psoriasis:

Sx: Hyperpigmented, thick, leathery, sharp margins, silvery scales
   Extensor surfaces

PE:

Dx: KOBNER phenomenon - AUSPITZ sign

_____

_____

_____

Tx:

Lichen Planus:

Sx: Itchy, flat-topped bumps,

PE: **P**urple, **P**apule, **P**olygonal, **P**ruritis, **P**lanar

Dx: KOEBNER phenomenon

    Wickham's Striae (white lines)

Tx:

_____

_____

_____

Lichen Simplex Chronicus: **Atopic dermatitis is precursor**

Sx: Lichenified plaques & excoriations, doesn't bleed when scratched

PE:

Dx:

Tx:

_____

_____

_____

Urticaria:

Sx: Allergic reaction - blanchable, pruritic, raised, erythematous or skin-colored papules, wheels or plaques on skin

PE: Darier's sign

Dx:

Tx:

_____

_____

_____

Diaper Dermatitis/Candida & Fungal Infection: **Irritant contact dermatitis**

Sx:

PE:

Dx:

_____   **Tx:**

_____

_____

Contact Dermatitis:

Sx: Well demarcated erythema, erosions, vesicles, pruritis, burning

PE:

Dx:

_____   **Tx:**

_____

_____

Folliculitis:

Sx: Erythematous papules or pustules involving hair follicles

PE:

Dx:

_____   **Tx:**

_____

_____

Nummular Eczema: **Coin shaped**

Sx: Mostly on extremities

PE:

Dx:

Tx:

Perioral Dermatitis:

Sx: Papulopustular, plaques, scales around mouth (vermillion border is spared)

PE:

Dx:

Tx:

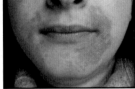

Dermatitis Herpetiform: **Associated w/celiac disease**

Sx: Autoimmune cutaneous eruption, gluten sensitivity

PE:

Dx: CBC and blood smear, tissue transglutaminase immunoglobulin A (tTg-IgA), skin biopsy, small bowel histology

_____   **Tx:**

_____

_____

Pressure Ulcer:

Sx: Exudate, foul odor, localized tenderness

PE:

Dx:

_____   **Tx:**

_____

_____

Seborrheic Dermatitis: **Cradle cap in infants**

Sx: Erythematous base. Yellow, greasy, scaly, patches, and crusted lesions

PE:

Dx:

_____   **Tx:**

_____

_____

Drug Eruptions:

Common causes: NSAIDs

Sx: Erythematous, edematous plaque that leaves behind *hyperpigmented* macule

PE:

Dx:

_____   Tx:

_____

_____

Vitiligo: **Hypopigmentation**

Co-occurring with pernicious anemia, autoimmune thyroiditis, Addison's, type 1 diabetes

Sx:

PE:

Dx: Wood's light fluorescence over the lesion

_____

_____

_____

Tx:

Melasma: **Hyperpigmentation**

Common causes: Estrongen, pregnancy, oral contraceptionn

Sx:

PE:

Dx:

_____   Tx:

_____

_____

Rosacea: **Rash, burns with certain foods (alcohol)**

Sx: Flushing, erythema, telangiectasis, papules and pustules

PE:

Dx:

_____

_____

_____

Tx:

Erysipelas: **Lower extremities = Strep pyogenes**
Face = Staph aureus

Sx: Abrupt onset, fever, chills, skin streaking with well defined margins (raised).

PE:

Dx:

_____

_____

_____

Tx:

Cellulitis: **Staph & strep**

Sx: Margins are NOT well demarcated, pain, erythema, warm, swelling

PE:

Dx:

_____

_____

_____

Tx:

Bullous Pemphigoid: **Chronic autoimmune, autoantibodies IgG**

Sx: Large fluid-filled bilsters

PE: Nikolsky

Dx:

_____   Tx:

_____

_____

Pemphigus Vulgaris: **Autoimmune**

Sx: Blistering of skin and/or mucosa

PX:

Dx: Skin biopsy with direct immunofluorescence

_____   Tx:

_____

_____

Simple Abscess: S. aureus – collection of pus within dermis and deeper tissue

Sx:

PE: Tender, erythematous, warm, fluctuant mass

Dx:

_____

_____

_____

Tx:

Furuncle: S. aureus – infection of hair follicle

Sx:

PE: Nodule or pustule that may have purulent drainage or discharge

Dx:

_____

_____

_____

Tx:

Carbuncle: S. aureus

Sx:

PE: Cluster of furuncles connected at subcutaneous layer

Dx:

_____

_____

_____

Tx:

Hidradenitis Suppurativa: Chronic follicular occlusive disease. Smoking correlates with severity of disease

Sx: Abscesses, sinus tracts, and scarring. Commonly in axillae, groin, and buttocks

PE:

Dx:

_____   Tx:

_____

_____

Pilonidal Disease:

Sx: Chronic follicle infection at the tailbone that contains hair and skin. Pain and swelling that comes and goes. Possible malodourous discharge

PE:

Dx:

_____   Tx:

_____

_____

PILONIDAL
CYST

Stevens-Johnson Syndrome (SJS): Skin & mucous membranes: 3-10% of body

Toxic-Epidermal Necrolysis (TEN): More than 30% of body

Sx: Rash, mucosal involvement

Prodrome: Flu-like symptoms

Painful, red or purplish rash that spreads, blisters

Associated with anticonvulsant meds, infection, antibiotic use, lupus, AIDS

PE:

Dx: Skin biopsy:

_____   Tx:

_____

_____

Scalded Skin Syndrome: Exfoliative toxin by S. aureus (spares mucous membranes)

Sx: Prodrome, fever, rapid progression of erythema in shin folds, pain

PE:

Dx: Bacterial culture

_____   **Tx:**

_____

_____

Drug Reaction with Eosinophilia and Systemic Symptoms (DRESS)

Common causes: Anticonvulsant (carbamazepine), allopurinol, sulfonamides, antibiotic

Sx: Skin eruption, fever, facial edema, visceral involvement, blood involvement

PE:

Dx:

_____   **Tx:**

_____

_____

Fungi or Dermatophytes

Epidermomycosis = Skin - Trichomycosis = Hair & hair follicles - Onychomycosis = Nails

Tinea Pedis: "Athlete's foot"

Sx:

PE:

Dx: Potassium hydroxide (KOH)

Tx:

_____

_____

_____

Tinea Cruris: "Jock itch"

Sx:

PE:

Dx: Potassium hydroxide (KOH)

Tx:

_____

_____

_____

Tinea Capitis (Pediculosis Capitis):

Sx: Patchy alopecia, scaling lesion with central clearing

PE:

Dx:

Tx:

_____

_____

_____

Tinea Corporis:

Sx: Well demarcated scaling plaques with central clearing

PE:

Dx: Potassium hydroxide (KOH) prep

_____   **Tx:**

_____

_____

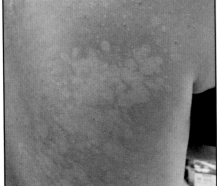

Tinea Versicolor: **Hypopigmentation caused by fungus (Malassezia furfur)**

Sx: Scaly patches on chest & trunk, may have mild itching

PE:

Dx:

_____   **Tx:**

_____

_____

Tinea Barbae: **Fungal infection caused by dermatophytes**

Sx:

PE:

Dx:

_____

_____   Tx:

_____

Onychomycosis:

Sx: Nail fungus causing thickened, brittle, crumbly nails

PE:

Dx: KOH prep or Periodic Acid-Schiff

_____

_____   Tx:

_____

Verrucae

Verruca Vulgaris (Common Wart):

Sx: Round, raised papule with tiny black dots

PE:

Dx:

_____   Tx:

_____

_____

Verruca Plana (Flat Wart):

Sx: Flat topped, slightly raised

PX:

Dx:

_____   Tx:

_____

_____

Verrucae Plantaris (Plantar Wart):

Sx:

PE: Hyperkeratotic debris with thrombosed capillaries

Dx:

_____

_____

_____

Tx: Salicylic acid, cryotherapy

Condyloma Acuminatum (Venereal Warts):

Risk Factors: Early age for intercourse, increased amount of sexual partners

Sx: Lesions 1-3 cm, sessile, papillomas that may coalesce into larger cauliflower like lesions

PE:

Dx:

_____

_____

_____

Tx:

Hair Loss (Alopecias)

Alopecia Areata: "Exclamation point hairs"

Risk Factors: Hashimoto's, Addison's, vitiligo, pernicious anemia

Sx: Smooth, non-scaring

PE:

Dx: Pull test, clinical

_____ Tx:

_____

_____

Traction Alopecia:

Sx:

PE:

Dx: Clinical

_____ Tx:

_____

_____

Telogen Effluvium: **Psychological or physiological stress**

Sx: Temporary thinning of hair

PE:

Dx:

_____   Tx:

_____

_____

Androgenic Alopecia: **Male pattern baldness**

Sx: Gradual receding hairline

PE:

Dx: Negative hair pull test, thyroid function, serum ferritin

_____   Tx:

_____

_____

Pediatric Derm Concerns

Erythema Infectiosum (Fifth Disease): **Parvo B19**

Sx: "Slapped cheek" spares nose and mouth. Lacy reticular rash on extremities that SPARES
   PALMS & SOLES

PE:

Dx:

_____

_____   Tx:

_____

Hand, Foot, and Mouth (Coxsackie Virus): **Respiratory droplets, summer & fall months**

Sx:

PE:

Dx: Viral culture, CBC

_____

_____   Tx:

_____

Measles (Rubeola):

Sx: 4 C's: Cough, coryza, conjunctivitis, cephalocaudal morbilliform rash

   Rash starts at hairline then moves to palms & soles of feet

   Rash lasts 7 days.

   Kolpik spots - small, erythematous spots on buccal mucosa with blue/white pale center, usually
   precedes rash by 1-2 days

PE:

Dx:

_____   Tx:

_____

_____

Rubella (German Measles):

Sx: Fever, maculopapular rash, postauricular lymphadenopathy
   3-day rash: pink, spotted maculopapular rash *first on face then to trunk & extremities*
   Pregnant women should avoid exposure

PE:

Dx:

_____   Tx:

_____

_____

Congenital Rubella: Microcephaly, ophthalmologist issues

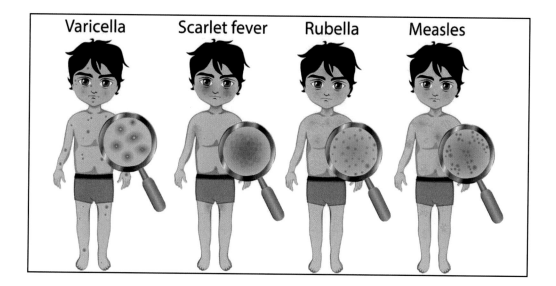

Impetigo: **S. aureus**

Sx: Honey crusted lesions

PE:

Dx:

_____ Tx:

_____

_____

Molluscum Contagiosum: **Poxvirus**

Sx: Pearly papules with umbilication

PE:

Dx:

_____ Tx:

_____

_____

Lice:

Sx: Scalp itching, visible eggs

PE:

Dx: Clinical

_____ Tx:

_____

Scabies:

Sx: Pruritic papules in an "s" shaped or linear pattern (burrows). Usually affects web spaces of hands, wrists, and waist. Itching that is worse at night

PE:

Dx:

_____

_____

_____

Tx:

Scabies

Erythemas

Erythema Multiforme: HSV (most common) and sulfa drugs

Sx: Target shaped, blanching, does not itch

PE:

Dx: CBC, HSV serology, PCR

Tx:

_____

_____

_____

Erythema Marginatum: Associated with rheumatic fever

Sx: Macule with central clearing that the spares face

PE:

Dx:

Tx:

_____

_____

_____

Erythema Nodosum:

Cause: Infection, autoimmune, medications, pregnancy, inflammatory conditions (Sarcoidosis, Crohn's)

Sx: Inflammatory nodules

PE:

Dx:

Tx:

_____

_____

_____

Spider Bites

Brown Recluse:

Sx: Necrotic wound

PE:

Dx:

_____   **Tx:**

_____

_____

Black Widow:

Sx: Neurologic manifestations

PE:

Dx:

_____   **Tx:**

_____

_____

Dermatologic Carcinomas

Actinic Keratosis: Most common cause sun exposure - PRE-CANCER

Sx: Single or multiple scaly macules or papules

PE:

Dx:

_____   Tx:

_____

_____

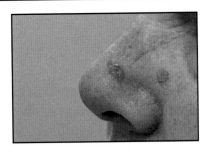

Squamous Cell Carcinoma: Actinic keratosis is precursor

Sx: Nonhealing lesion, may bleed. Location: Sun-exposed areas

PE:

Dx:

_____   Tx:

_____

_____

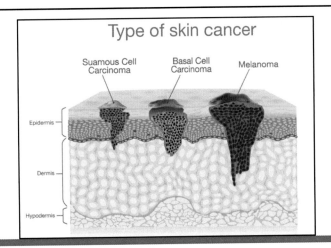

Type of skin cancer

Suamous Cell Carcinoma   Basal Cell Carcinoma   Melanoma

Epidermis

Dermis

Hypodermis

Melanoma:

Sx: Asymmetry, border irregularity, color variations, diameter > 6mm

PE:

Dx:

_____

_____

_____

Tx:

ABCDE
(the first signs of a melanoma)

Asymmetry
Borders
Color
Diameter
Evolving

Diameter
(about 6 mm)

Asymmetry

Borders
(irregular or jagged)

Evolving
(change in size,
shape, color or elevation)

Color
(multiple colors: brown,
black, red, white or blue)

Basal Cell Carcinoma: **Most common skin cancer**

Sx: Pearly nodule, "rolled" raised edge, telangiectasis, non-healing scabs,
     ulcerated center with pearly heaped edges

PE:

Dx:

_____   Tx:

_____

_____

Acne

Acne:

Sx: Uninflamed blackheads, pustules, large erythematous and tender bumps

PE:

Dx:

_____   **Tx:**

_____

_____

TYPES OF ACNE

Acne Vulgaris:

Sx:

PE: Comedones, inflamed nodules

Dx: Clinical

_____   **Tx:**

_____

_____

Misc. Derm

Seborrheic Keratosis:

Sx: Yellow or light to dark brown lesions, raised, waxy, painless

PE:

Dx:

_____

_____   Tx:

_____

Erythrasma:

Sx: Sharply delineated, dry, brown, scaling patches (axillae, genitocrural creases)

PE:

Dx:

_____

_____

_____

Tx:

Pityriasis Rosea: Self-limiting

Sx: Herald Patch, central clearing with Christmas tree distribution
(Langer's lines), salmon-colored patches

PE:

Dx:

_____

_____

_____

Tx:

Dog Bite:

Sx: Laceration

PE:

Dx: Clinical

_____   **Tx:**

_____

_____

Cat Bite: Pasteurella most common bacteria

Sx: Laceration, puncture wounds

PE:

Dx: Clinical

_____   **Tx:**

_____

_____

Cherry Angioma:

Sx: Flat, small, red

PE:

Dx:

_____   Tx:

_____

_____

Solar Lentigo: **Liver spots**

Sx:

PE:

Dx: Skin biopsy

_____   Tx:

_____

_____

Sebaceous Cyst: **Blocked gland or duct**

Sx: Can range in size

PE:

Dx:

_____   Tx:

_____

_____

Keloids: **Abnormal scarring**

Sx:

PE:

Dx: Clinical

_____   **Tx:**

_____

_____

Lipoma:

Sx: Slow growing and usually harmless

PE:

Dx: X-ray, MRI, or biopsy to rule out other causes

_____   **Tx:**

_____

_____

Burns

Rule of 9's

*Paronychia: **In MSK***

*Roseola (6th disease) (Herpesvirus 6 or 7): **In ID***

*Felon: **In MSK***

*Genital Herpes: **In ID***

*Erythema Migrans (Lyme Disease): **In ID***

Medications

_____: MOA = _____

Indication(s)=_____

Side Effects = _____

Types/ Examples = _____

_____

_____

_____: MOA = _____

Indication(s)=_____

Side Effects = _____

Types/ Examples = _____

_____

_____

_____: MOA = _____

Indication(s)=_____

Side Effects = _____

Types/ Examples = _____

_____

_____

_____: MOA = _____

Indication(s)=_____

Side Effects = _____

Types/ Examples = _____

_____

_____

_____: MOA = _____

Indication(s)=_____

Side Effects = _____

Types/ Examples = _____

_____

Medications

_____: MOA = _____

Indication(s)=_____

Side Effects = _____

Types/ Examples = _____

_____

_____

_____: MOA = _____

Indication(s)=_____

Side Effects = _____

Types/ Examples = _____

_____

_____

_____: MOA = _____

Indication(s)=_____

Side Effects = _____

Types/ Examples = _____

_____

_____

_____: MOA = _____

Indication(s)=_____

Side Effects = _____

Types/ Examples = _____

_____

_____

_____: MOA = _____

Indication(s)=_____

Side Effects = _____

Types/ Examples = _____

_____

Endocrinology

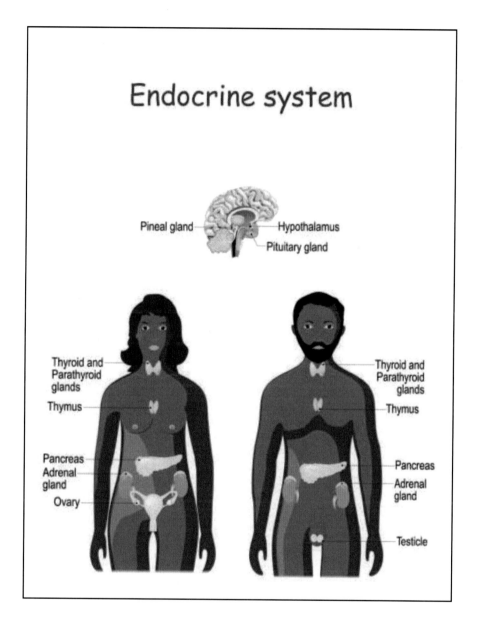

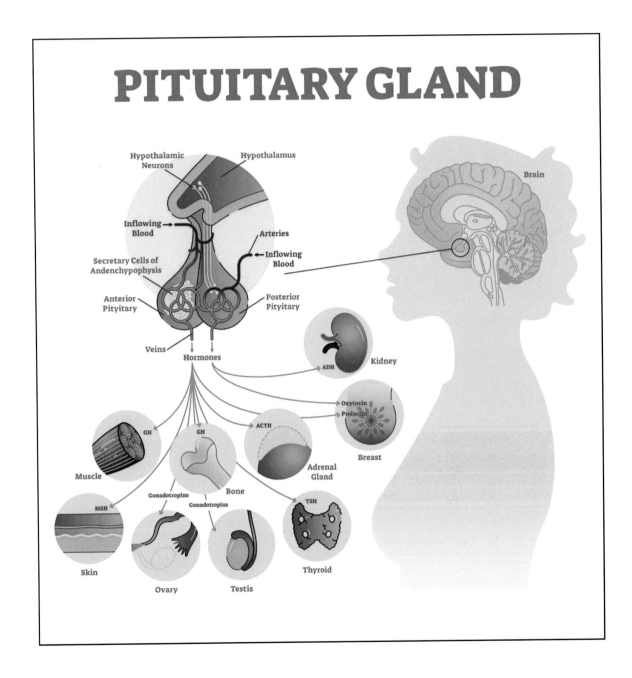

Thyroid Disorders

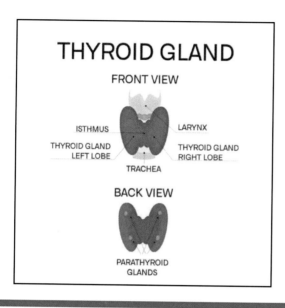

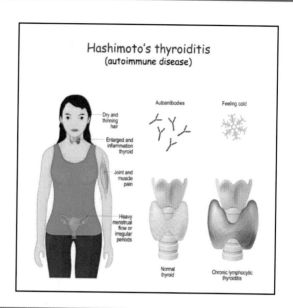

Hypothyroidism:

Hashimoto's:

Sx: Cold intolerance, dry skin, fatigue, constipation, hair loss

PE:

Dx: Increase TSH, decrease T3 & T4, + anti-thyroid peroxidase AB, + anti-thyroglobin Ab

_____   **Tx:**

_____

_____

Myxedema: Extreme form of hypothyroidism

Sx: Bradycardia, hypothermia, hypoglycemia

PE:

Dx:

_____   **Tx:**

_____

_____

Hyperthyroidism:

Sx: Heat intolerance, weight loss, hyperactivity, diarrhea, tachycardia

PE:

Dx: Decreased TSH

_____   Tx:

_____

_____

Graves' Disease: **Most common cause of hyperthyroidism**

Sx:

PE:

Dx: Decreased TSH, increased T3 & T4

_____

_____

_____

Tx:

Graves' disease symptoms: Exophthalmos, Goiter, Sweating, Arrhythmia and tachycardia, Headache, Weight loss, Nervousness, Emotional instability, Nausea and diarrhea, Oligomenorrhea (in female), Tremor, Muscle weakness

Thyroid Storm: **Extreme form of hyperthyroidism**

Sx: Palpitations, high fever, nausea, vomiting, psychosis, tremors

PE:

Dx:

_____   Tx:

_____

_____

Thyroid Nodule:

Sx: Most often asymptomatic

PE:

Dx: Fine needle aspiration with biopsy

_____   Tx:

_____

_____

Thyroid Cancer:

Papillary (most common, good prognosis) _____

_____

Follicular (good prognosis) _____

_____

Medullary (MEN2, poor prognosis) _____

_____

Anaplastic (worst prognosis) _____

_____

Sx:

PE:

Dx:

_____   Tx:

_____

_____

Thyroid Medications:
Hyperthyroid:

Methimazole:

PTU:

Propranolol:

Iodides:

Radioactive Iodine:

Hypothyroid:

Levothyroxine:

Parathyroid Disorders

Low serum Ca - Parathyroid glands - PTH - bones & kidneys

PTH at bones stimulates osteoclasts to break down bone

PTH at kidneys stimulates calcitriol (vit D) release – small intestines absorb more Ca

---

Hyperparathyroidism:

Sx: Stones, bones, moans, groans (kidney stones, bone pain, myalgia, fatigue)

PE:

Dx:

_____   Tx:

_____

_____

Hypoparathyroidism:

Most common cause: Thyroidectomy

Sx: Tetany, spasms, cramps

PE:

Dx:

_____   Tx:

_____

_____

Adrenal Gland Disorders

Hypothalamus - CRH – Anterior pit - ACTH – Adrenal cortex – Cortisol -

Adrenal medulla - Catecholamines (EPI & NorEPI)

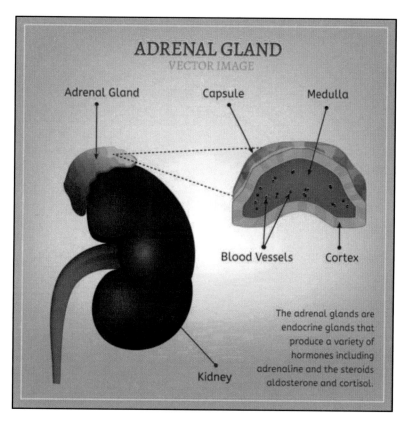

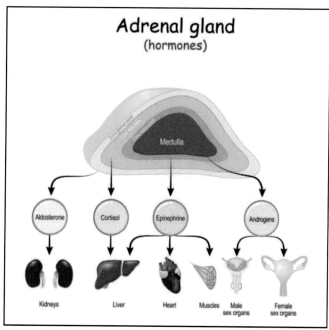

Cushing's Disease/Syndrome:

Causes:

Sx:

PE: Moon face, buffalo hump

Dx:

_____   Tx:

_____

_____

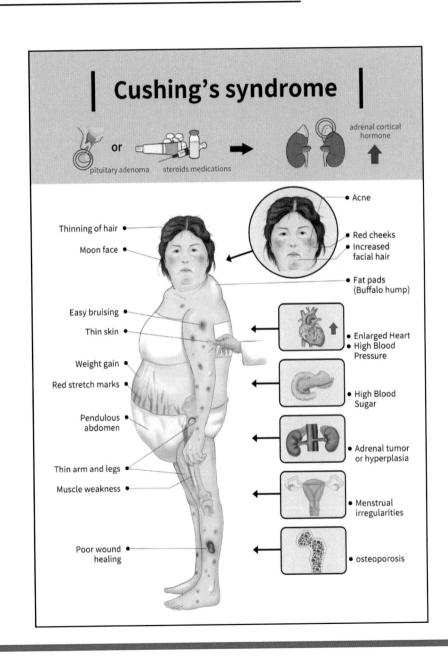

Addison's Disease:

Causes:

Sx:

PE: Hyperpigmentation (JFK)

Dx:

_____   **Tx:**

_____

_____

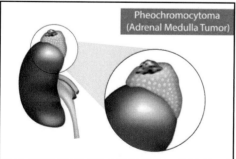

Pheochromocytoma: Adrenal catecholamine secreting tumor

Sx:

PE: Resistant hypertension, palpitations, headaches, excessive sweating

Dx:

_____   **Tx:**

_____

_____

Pituitary Gland Disorders

Syndrome of Inappropriate Antidiuretic Hormone (SIADH):

Causes: Pituitary trauma, tumor (lung or GI)

Sx: Symptoms of hyponatremia, concentrated urine

PE:

Dx:

_____   **Tx:**

_____

_____

Diabetes Insipidus (DI):

Central DI: Pituitary/hypothalamus (decreased ADH production)

Sx:

PE:

Dx: Fluid deprivation test = continued dilute urine. Desmopressin stimulation = decreased urine output and increased urine osmolality

Nephrogenic DI: Kidney (insensitivity to ADH)

Sx:

PE:

Dx: Fluid deprivation test = continued dilute urine. Desmopressin stimulation = continued dilute urine

_____   **Tx:**

_____

_____

Acromegaly (Adults)/Giantism (Children):
Most common cause: Pituitary adenoma

Sx:

PE:

Dx: Increase in insulin-like growth factor 1 (IGF-1)

_____   **Tx:**

_____

_____

Dwarfism: **Growth hormone deficiency**

Sx:

PE:

Dx:

_____   **Tx:**

_____

_____

Prolactinoma:

Sx: Breast enlargement, amenorrhea, decreased libido

PE:

Dx:

_____   **Tx:**

_____

_____

Hyperprolactinemia: Most common cause is prolactinoma

Increased prolactin levels inhibit gonadotropin releasing hormone which causes a decrease in FSH/LH

Sx:

PE:

Dx:

_____   Tx:

_____

_____

Hypogonadism:

Sx:

PE:

Dx: Low testosterone

_____   Tx:

_____

_____

Pituitary Adenoma:

Sx:

PE:

Dx: Pituitary MRI

_____   Tx:

_____

_____

Diabetes Mellitus

Insulin = hormone secreted by pancreatic B cells (allows glucose into cells)

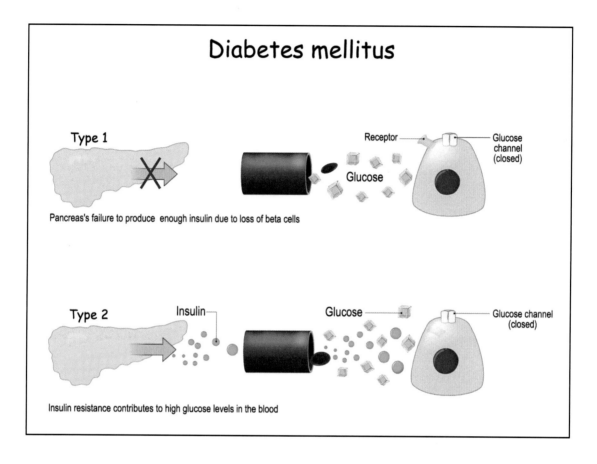

Diabetes Mellitus I: **Autoimmune**

Sx: Polyuria, polydipsia, polyphagia

PE:

Dx:

_____   **Tx:**

_____

_____

Diabetes Mellitus ll:

Sx:

PE:

Dx: Hb A1C > 6.5%, fasting glucose > 125 mg/dL, random glucose > 200 mg/dL

_____   **Tx:**

_____

_____

Diabetic Ketoacidosis (DKA): **Complication often associated with type I diabetes**

Sx:

PE: Fruity breath

Dx:

_____   **Tx:**

_____

_____

Hyperosmolar Hyperglycemic Syndrome (HHS): **Complication of type II diabetes**

Sx:

PE:

Dx: Hyperglycemia (glucose > 600mg/dL) and hyperosmolality (> 320 mOsm/kg)

_____   **Tx:**

_____

_____

Hypoglycemia:

Sx: Nausea, confusion, sweating, palpitations, hunger

PE:

Dx:

_____   **Tx:**

_____

_____

Metabolic Syndrome (Including Insulin Resistance):

Sx: Skin tags, acanthosis nigricans, central abdominal obesity

PE:

Dx:

_____   **Tx:**

_____

_____

Gynecomastia:

Sx: Enlargement of breast tissue

PE:

Dx:

_____   **Tx:**

_____

_____

Multiple Endocrine Neoplasia (MEN): Hereditary tumor syndromes with distinct patterns of organ involvement

Sx:

PE:

Dx:

_____   **Tx:**

_____

_____

Diabetes Medications

Insulin:

MOA = _____

Indication(s) = _____

Side Effects = _____

Types/ Examples = _____

Biguanides - Metformin:

MOA = _____

Indication(s) = _____

Side Effects = _____

Types/ Examples = _____

Sulfonylureas:

MOA = _____

Indication(s) = _____

Side Effects = _____

Types/ Examples = _____

Meglitinides:

MOA = _____

Indication(s) = _____

Side Effects = _____

Types/ Examples = _____

Thiazolidinediones:

MOA = _____

Indication(s) = _____

Side Effects = _____

Types/ Examples = _____

Alpha - Glucosidase Inhibitor:

MOA = _____

Indication(s) = _____

Side Effects = _____

Types/ Examples = _____

GLP - 1 Agonists:

MOA = _____

Indication(s) = _____

Side Effects = _____

Types/ Examples = _____

DDP - 4 Antagonists:

MOA = _____

Indication(s) = _____

Side Effects = _____

Types/ Examples = _____

Medications

_____: MOA = _____

Indication(s)=_____

Side Effects = _____

Types/ Examples = _____

_____

_____

_____: MOA = _____

Indication(s)=_____

Side Effects = _____

Types/ Examples = _____

_____

_____

_____: MOA = _____

Indication(s)=_____

Side Effects = _____

Types/ Examples = _____

_____

_____

_____: MOA = _____

Indication(s)=_____

Side Effects = _____

Types/ Examples = _____

_____

_____

_____: MOA = _____

Indication(s)=_____

Side Effects = _____

Types/ Examples = _____

_____

Medications

_____: MOA = _____

Indication(s)=_____

Side Effects = _____

Types/ Examples = _____

_____

_____

_____: MOA = _____

Indication(s)=_____

Side Effects = _____

Types/ Examples = _____

_____

_____

_____: MOA = _____

Indication(s)=_____

Side Effects = _____

Types/ Examples = _____

_____

_____

_____: MOA = _____

Indication(s)=_____

Side Effects = _____

Types/ Examples = _____

_____

_____

_____: MOA = _____

Indication(s)=_____

Side Effects = _____

Types/ Examples = _____

_____

Psychiatric
Depressive Disorders

Major Depressive Disorder: SIEGCAPS > 2 weeks

Sx:

PE:

Dx: DSM V

Tx:

_____

_____

_____

Persistent Depressive Disorder (PDD) "Dysthymia": Symptoms > 2 years with no more than 2 months no symptoms

Sx:

PE:

Dx: DSM V

Tx:

_____

_____

_____

Premenstrual Dysphoric Disorder (PMDD): Symptoms occurring 1-2 weeks before menses (luteal phase), relieved within 2-3 days of the onset of menses + 7 days no symptoms during follicular phase

Sx: Irritability, labile mood, anger

PE:

Dx: DSM V

Tx:

_____

_____

_____

Seasonal Affect Disorder (SAD): Winter months, less sunlight

Sx: Persistent low mood, anhedonia, low energy

PE:

Dx: DSM V

_____   Tx:

_____

_____

Adjustment Disorder: Symptoms of emotion and behavior occurring within 3 months of a stressor

Sx: Impairment of functioning

PE:

Dx: DSM V

_____   Tx:

_____

_____

Bipolar Disorders

Bipolar I: At least 1 manic episode with or without depression, must have 1 manic episode lasting > 1 week

Sx: DIGFAST

PE:

Dx: DSM V

_____   Tx:

_____

_____

Bipolar II: Major depressive disorder + 1 or more episode(s) of hypomania lasting 4-6 days

Sx:

PE:

Dx: DSM V

_____   Tx:

_____

_____

Cyclothymic Disorder: At least 2 years of hypomanic and depressive episodes that do not meet criteria for Bipolar I or Major Depressive Disorder

Sx:

PE:

Dx: DSM V

_____   Tx:

_____

_____

Anxiety Disorders

Generalized Anxiety Disorder (GAD): Anxiety symptoms for 6+ months

Sx: Restlessness, Irritability, sleep disturbance

PE:

Dx: DSM V

_____   Tx:

_____

_____

Panic Attack: Sense of impending doom

Sx:

PE:

Dx: DSM V

_____   Tx:

_____

_____

Panic Disorder: 2+ panic attacks followed by > 1 month of worry about recurrence

Sx: Anxiety, palpitations

PE:

Dx: DSM V

_____   Tx:

_____

_____

Specific Phobia: > 6 months

Sx: Persistent anxiety or fear of a specific situation or thing

PE:

Dx: DSM V

_____   Tx:

_____

_____

Social Anxiety Disorder: > 6 months

Sx: Intense, persistent fear of social situations or performance

PE:

Dx: DSM V

_____   Tx:

_____

_____

Agoraphobia: Fear of enclosed spaces, crowds, or leaving one's home > 6 months

Sx:

PE:

Dx: DSM V

_____   Tx:

_____

_____

Obsessive Compulsive Disorder: > 1 hour per day

Sx: Obsessions: Intrusive, recurrent thoughts that cause anxiety or stress
   Compulsions: Repetitive behaviors or mental acts to relieve anxiety

PE:

Dx: DSM V

_____   Tx:

_____

_____

Post-Traumatic Stress Disorder (PTSD): Trauma exposure, flashbacks > 1 month

Sx: Nightmares, flashbacks, sleep problems, hypervigilance, avoidance of thoughts, feelings, & memories

PE:

Dx: DSM V

_____   Tx:

_____

_____

Acute Stress Disorder: Same as PTSD, but shorter time frame < 1 month

Sx:

PE:

Dx: DSM V

_____   Tx:

_____

_____

Trichotillomania: **Hair pulling disorder**

Sx: Pulling out of one's hair with repeated attempts to decrease or stop hair pulling

PE:

Dx: DSM V

_____   **Tx:**

_____

_____

Hoarding Disorder:

Sx: Difficulty parting with possessions that congest and clutter active living areas

PE:

Dx: DSM V

_____   **Tx:**

_____

_____

Psychotic Disorders

Delusional Disorder: > 1 month with 1 or more delusions without significant impairment in functioning

Sx: 1 or more delusions

PE:

Dx: DSM V

_____   Tx:

_____

_____

Schizophrenia: 2 or more positive symptoms > 6 months

Positive Sx: Hallucinations, delusions, or disorganized speech
Negative Sx: Blunted affect, anhedonia

PE:

Dx: DSM V

_____   Tx:

_____

_____

Brief Psychotic Disorder: Psychotic symptoms for 1 day to 1 month

Sx: Psychotic symptoms

PE:

Dx: DSM V

_____   Tx:

_____

_____

Schizophreniform: 1 month - 6 months

Sx: Same as schizophrenia

PE:

Dx: DSM V

_____ **Tx:**

_____

_____

Schizoaffective Disorder:

Sx: Schizophrenia symptoms + mood symptoms

PE:

Dx: DSM V

_____ **Tx:**

_____

_____

Personality Disorders
Cluster A (The Weird)

Paranoid: Suspicious and distrusting of others

Sx: Suspects others are exploiting them

PE:

Dx: DSM V

_____   Tx:

_____

_____

Schizoid: Detachment from social relationships

Sx: No desire for close relationships

PE:

Dx: DSM V

_____   Tx:

_____

_____

Schizotypal:

Sx: Odd beliefs or magical thinking

PE:

Dx: DSM V

_____   Tx:

_____

_____

Cluster B (The Wild)

Antisocial: > 18 years old, behaviors deviate from societal norms, values, and laws

Sx: Non-conforming to social norms, irritable, irresponsible, lack of remorse

PE:

Dx: DSM V

_____   Tx:

_____

_____

Histrionic: Begins early adulthood, variety of settings

Sx: Emotional, dramatic, attention seeking

PE:

Dx: DSM V

_____   Tx:

_____

_____

Borderline:

Sx: Unstable relationships, impulsive, mood swings, recurrent suicidal behaviors, gestures or threats

PE:

Dx: DSM V

_____   Tx:

_____

_____

Narcissistic:

Sx: Big ego, no empathy, sensitive to failure, exploit others, grandiose sense of self-importance

PE:

Dx: DSM V

_____   Tx:

_____

_____

Cluster C (The Worried)

Avoidant:

Sx: Afraid of rejection, social inhibition

PE:

Dx: DSM V

_____

_____   Tx:

_____

Dependent:

Sx: Afraid of abandonment, passive, low self-esteem, submissive and clingy behaviors

PE:

Dx: DSM V

_____

_____   Tx:

_____

Obsessive Compulsive Personality Disorder:

Sx: Control, rigid, perfectionistic, expects others to meet increased standards

PE:

Dx: DSM V

_____

_____   Tx:

_____

Somatic Disorders

Somatic Symptom Disorder: 1 or more somatic symptoms + anxiety with NO CAUSE > 6 months

Sx: High levels of anxiety about one's health

PE:

Dx: DSM V

_____   Tx:

_____

_____

Illness Anxiety Disorder: Hypochondriac with anxiety about health > 6 months

Sx:

PE:

Dx: DSM V

_____   Tx:

_____

_____

Conversion Disorder: Neuro symptoms without having a neuro or medical condition. Negative EEG and labs

Sx: Intermittent paralysis, bizarre movements

PE:

Dx: DSM V

_____   Tx:

_____

_____

Factitious Disorder: **Consciously has false symptoms to play sick role**

Sx: Person presents themselves as injured or ill

PE:

Dx: DSM V

_____   Tx:

_____

_____

Factitious Disorder by Proxy: **Consciously puts false symptoms onto others**

Sx: Perpetrator, presents victim (most often their child) as injured or ill

PE:

Dx: DSM V

_____   Tx:

_____

_____

Malingering: **Intentional false symptoms for external gain**

Sx: Exaggeration or fabrication of mental or physical symptoms for gain

PE:

Dx: DSM V

_____   Tx:

_____

_____

Pseudocyesis: **False belief that one is pregnant**

Sx:

PE:

Dx: DSM V

_____   Tx:

_____

_____

Developmental Psych and Behavioral Disorders

Attention Deficit Hyperactivity Disorder (ADHD):

Sx: Difficulty paying attention, impulsivity, and hyperactivity

PE:

Dx: DSM V

_____   **Tx:**

_____

_____

Inattention:

Hyperactivity and Impulsivity:

Combined Type:

Autism Spectrum Disorder (ASD): **Spectrum of developmental disorders**

Sx: Social interaction problems, impaired communication, restricted, repetitive patterns of behavior, interests or activities

PE:

Dx: DSM V

_____   **Tx:**

_____

_____

Conduct Disorder: < 18 years old, may progress to antisocial personality disorder

Sx: Violates rights of others, may hurt animals, lacks remorse

PE:

Dx: DSM V

_____   **Tx:**

_____

_____

Oppositional Defiant Disorder (ODD):

Sx: Easily annoyed, often angry, spiteful, deliberately annoys

PE:

Dx: DSM V

_____   **Tx:**

_____

_____

Disruptive Mood Dysregulation Disorder:

Sx: Temper outburst, out of proportion to situation or provoking event, irritable mood between outbursts

PE:

Dx: DSM V

_____   **Tx:**

_____

_____

Eating Disorders

Anorexia Nervosa: Preoccupation with body weight & image

Restrictive type Sx:

Dx: DSM V

Binge eating and purging type Sx:

Dx: DSM V

_____   Tx:

_____

_____

Bulimia Nervosa: Binging and inappropriate compensatory behaviors (usually purging)

Sx:

PE: Russell's sign

Dx: DSM V

_____   Tx:

_____

_____

Binge Eating Disorder: Recurrent episodes of binge eating - at least weekly for 3 months

Sx:

PE:

Dx: DSM V

_____   Tx:

_____

_____

Body Dysmorphia:

Sx: Preoccupation with defects or flaws in one's personal appearance

PE:

Dx: DSM V

_____   Tx:

_____

_____

Sleep Disorders

Narcolepsy: Episodes occurring at least 3 times per week for 3+ months

Sx: Chronic daytime sleepiness, cataplexy

PE:

Dx: DSM V

_____   Tx:

_____

_____

Hypersomnolence: Excessive sleepiness

Sx: Prolonged sleep episodes longer than 9 hours per day

PE:

Dx: DSM V

_____   Tx:

_____

_____

Insomnia:

Sx: Difficulty initiating sleep, difficulty maintaining sleep, waking up early

PE:

Dx: DSM V

_____   Tx:

_____

_____

Nightmare Disorders:

Sx:

PE:

Dx: DSM V

_____   **Tx:**

_____

_____

Parasomnias

Sleepwalking:

Sx: Walking around while sleeping

PE:

Dx: DSM V

_____   **Tx:**

_____

_____

Sleep Terrors:

Sx: Abrupt arousal from sleep, sometimes with panic and screaming

PE:

Dx: DSM V

_____   **Tx:**

_____

_____

Drug Abuse/Dependence

Tobacco Use Dependance:

Sx:

PE:

Dx: DSM V

_____   **Tx:**

_____

_____

Nicotine withdrawal:

Sx:

Alcohol Use/Dependance:

Sx: Increased CNS activity, seizures, hallucinations, delirium tremens

PE:

Dx: DSM V

_____   **Tx:**

_____

_____

Alcohol withdrawal:

Sx:

Opioid Use/Dependance:

Sx: Pupillary constriction, altered mental status, respiratory depression

PE:

Dx: DSM V

_____   **Tx:**

_____

_____

Opioid withdrawal:

Sx:

Cocaine Intoxication:

Sx: Tremor, flushing, hyperthermia, pupillary dilation, cold sweats

PE:

Dx: DSM V

_____   **Tx:**

_____

_____

Cocaine withdrawal:

Sx:

PCP Intoxication:

Sx: Impulsivity, fear, rage, psychosis, delirium, hallucinations

PE:

Dx: DSM V

_____   **Tx:**

_____

_____

PCP withdrawal

Sx:

Marijuana Intoxication:

Sx: Euphoria, giddiness, anxiety, disinhibition, intensification of sensory experiences, cotton mouth

PE:

Dx: DSM V

_____   **Tx:**

_____

_____

Marijuana withdrawal:

Sx:

Dissociative Disorders

Dissociative Identity Disorder (DID):

Sx: 2+ distinct personality states

PE:

Dx: DSM V

_____   Tx:

_____

_____

Dissociative Amnesia:

Sx: Difficulty recalling autobiographical information, usually related to trauma or stress

PE:

Dx: DSM V

_____   Tx:

_____

_____

Dissociative Fugue:

Sx: Amnesia + travel

PE:

Dx: DSM V

_____   Tx:

_____

_____

Depersonalization/Derealization Disorder:

Sx: Unreality, detachment, feeling like an outside observer

PE:

Dx: DMS V

_____   Tx:

_____

_____

Types of Abuse

Child Physical Abuse: **Non-accidental physical injury to a child**

Sx: Bruising, fractures, death

PE:

Dx: DSM V

_____   Tx:

_____

_____

Child Neglect:

Sx: Deprivation of age-appropriate needs resulting in physical or psychological harm

PE:

Dx: DSM V

_____   Tx:

_____

_____

Sexual Abuse:

Sx:

PE:

Dx: DSM V

_____   Tx:

_____

_____

Intimate Partner Abuse:

Sx:

PE:

Dx: DSM V

_____   Tx:

_____

_____

Sexual Disorders

Exhibitionistic Disorder:

Sx: Sexual arousal from exposing oneself

PE:

Dx: DSM V

_____

_____   Tx:

_____

Fetishistic Disorder:

Sx: Sexual arousal from nonliving objects or nongenital body parts

PE:

Dx: DSM V

_____

_____   Tx:

_____

Frotteuristic Disorder:

Sx: Sexual arousal from touching or rubbing up against a non-consenting person

PE:

Dx: DSM V

_____

_____   Tx:

_____

Pedophile Disorder:

Sx: Sexual fantasies, urges involving prepubescent child or children

PE:

Dx: DSM V

_____   **Tx:**

_____

_____

Sexual Masochism Disorder:

Sx: Sexual arousal in response to pain or humiliation

PE:

Dx: DSM V

_____   **Tx:**

_____

_____

Sexual Sadism Disorder:

Sx: Sexual arousal from the physical or psychological suffering of another person

PE:

Dx: DSM V

_____   **Tx:**

_____

_____

Voyeuristic Disorder:

Sx: Sexual arousal from watching naked, unsuspecting persons

PE:

Dx: DSM V

_____   **Tx:**

_____

_____

Misc. Psych Disorders

Grief Reaction: Severe symptoms > 1 year

Sx:

PE:

Dx:

_____   Tx:

_____

_____

Suicide:

Sx:

PE:

Dx:

_____   Tx:

_____

_____

Serotonin Syndrome: Life threatening, increased serotonin within 6-24 hours of initiation or change in serotonergic drugs

Sx:

PE:

Dx:

_____   Tx:

_____

_____

Neuroleptic Malignant Syndrome: Life threatening, complication of treatment with antipsychotics

Sx: Hyperthermia, altered mental status

PE:

Dx:

_____   Tx:

_____

_____

Tourette Syndrome:

Sx: "Tics" repeated sounds, movements, or twitches

PE:

Dx:

_____   Tx:

_____

_____

Postpartum Depression: In Women's Health

Medications

_____: MOA = _____

Indication(s)=_____

Side Effects = _____

Types/ Examples = _____

_____

_____

_____: MOA = _____

Indication(s)=_____

Side Effects = _____

Types/ Examples = _____

_____

_____

_____: MOA = _____

Indication(s)=_____

Side Effects = _____

Types/ Examples = _____

_____

_____

_____: MOA = _____

Indication(s)=_____

Side Effects = _____

Types/ Examples = _____

_____

_____

_____: MOA = _____

Indication(s)=_____

Side Effects = _____

Types/ Examples = _____

_____

Medications

_____: MOA = _____

Indication(s)=_____

Side Effects = _____

Types/ Examples = _____

_____

_____

_____: MOA = _____

Indication(s)=_____

Side Effects = _____

Types/ Examples = _____

_____

_____

_____: MOA = _____

Indication(s)=_____

Side Effects = _____

Types/ Examples = _____

_____

_____

_____: MOA = _____

Indication(s)=_____

Side Effects = _____

Types/ Examples = _____

_____

_____

_____: MOA = _____

Indication(s)=_____

Side Effects = _____

Types/ Examples = _____

_____

Women's Health
Menstruation Disorders

Amenorrhea: Transient or permanent absence of menstrual flow
Primary amenorrhea:

Sx: No menses by age 15

PE:

Dx:

_____   **Tx:**

_____

_____

Causes: Hypothalamic, pituitary insufficiency, low FSH & LH, anorexia

Turner Syndrome: XO karyotype

Sx:

PE: Webbed neck, broad chest

Dx: High FSH

_____   **Tx:**

_____

_____

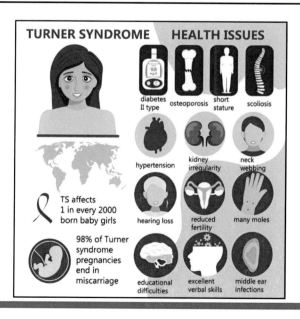

Androgen Insensitivity:

Sx:

PE: Breast development only

Dx: High testosterone

_____   **Tx:**

_____

_____

Müllerian Agenesis:

Sx:

PE: Secondary sex characteristics, no uterus

Dx:

_____   **Tx:**

_____

_____

Imperforate Hymen: **Blocked vaginal opening**

Sx: Can block menstrual flow

PE:

Dx:

_____   **Tx:**

_____

_____

Secondary Amenorrhea:

Sx: Absence of menses for 3+ cycles after previously having normal periods

PE:

Dx:

_____

_____

_____

Tx:

Causes: Hypothyroid, prolactinoma

Asherman Syndrome: Amenorrhea after an intrauterine procedure (e.g., D&C, or complication from procedural surgery)

Sx:

PE: No specific findings

Dx:

_____

_____

_____

Tx:

Dysfunctional Uterine Bleeding

Polymenorrhagia: Menses < 21 days   Tx:

_____

_____

Menorrhagia: Prolonged bleeding (> 7 days or > 80 mL) during menses   Tx:

_____

_____

Metrorrhagia: Uterine bleeding that occurs more frequently and   Tx:
irregularly between menses

_____

_____

Menometrorrhagia: Increased blood loss during menses as well as frequent   Tx:
and irregular bleeding between menses

_____

_____

Oligomenorrhea: Long intervals between menses > 35 days   Tx:

_____

_____

Dx:

Painful Uterine Bleeding

Dysmenorrhea: Pain peaks 24 hours after the onset of menses and subsides after 2-3 days   Tx:

Primary Dysmenorrhea: No organic cause - excessive prostaglandins   Tx:

Secondary Dysmenorrhea: Painful menstruation caused by clinically identifiable cause
Etiology: Endometriosis, adenomyosis, polyps, fibroids, PID, IUD, adhesions, tumors

Tx:

Dx:

Menstruation

Follicular (Proliferative) Phase: Days 0-14: Estrogen prominent
GnRH (from hypothalamus) stimulates FSH and LH (from anterior pituitary) which then triggers ovulation

_____

_____

_____

_____

_____

_____

_____

Ovulation:
GnRH (from hypothalamus) stimulates FSH and LH (from anterior pituitary) which then triggers ovulation

_____

_____

_____

_____

_____

_____

_____

Luteal (Secretory) Phase: Days 15-28: Progesterone prominent
After ovulation, the follicle becomes the corpus luteum, which secretes progesterone and provides negative feedback to FSH & LH

_____

_____

_____

_____

_____

_____

_____

MENSTRUAL CYCLE

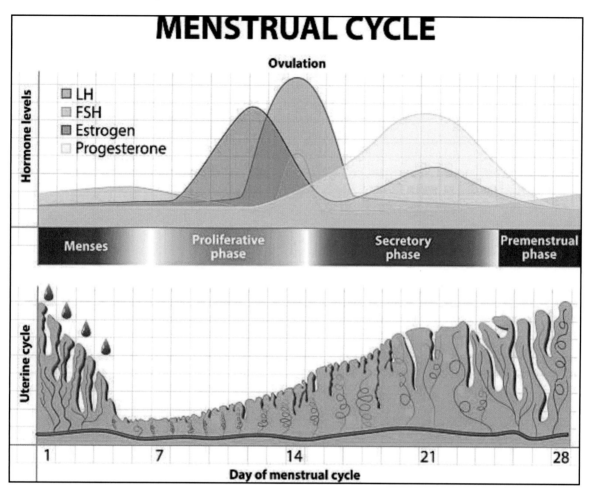

Ovulation

Hormone levels

- LH
- FSH
- Estrogen
- Progesterone

| Menses | Proliferative phase | Secretory phase | Premenstrual phase |

Uterine cycle

1   7   14   21   28

Day of menstrual cycle

MENSTRUAL CYCLE

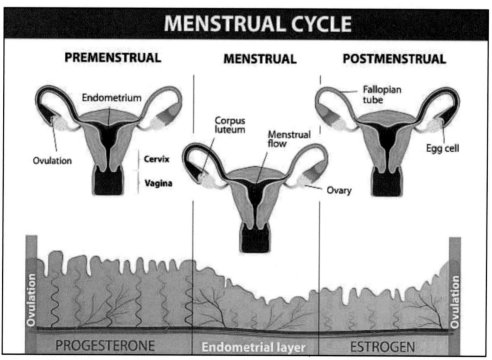

PREMENSTRUAL   **MENSTRUAL**   **POSTMENSTRUAL**

Endometrium

Corpus luteum

Menstrual flow

Fallopian tube

Ovulation

Cervix

Vagina

Egg cell

Ovary

Ovulation

PROGESTERONE   Endometrial layer   ESTROGEN

Ovulation

Premenstrual Syndrome (PMS):

Sx: Bloating & irritability during luteal phase

PE:

Dx:

_____   **Tx:**

_____

_____

Menopause: 12 or more months of amenorrhea

Sx: Hot flashes, night sweats, irritability, vaginal dryness

PE:

Dx: Labs: Increased FSH, decreased estradiol

_____   **Tx:**

_____

_____

Atrophic Vaginitis: Pale, atrophic epithelium with flattened rugae

Sx: Vaginal dryness, burning, possible dysuria

PE:

Dx:

_____   **Tx:**

_____

_____

Birth Control

Hormonal IUD:

MOA = _____

Indication(s)= _____

Side Effects= _____

Types/ Examples= _____

Non-Hormonal IUD:

MOA = _____

Indication(s)= _____

Side Effects= _____

Types/ Examples= _____

Nexplanon:

MOA = _____

Indication(s)= _____

Side Effects= _____

Types/ Examples= _____

Depo-Provera:

MOA = _____

Indication(s)= _____

Side Effects= _____

Types/ Examples= _____

Vaginal Ring:

MOA = _____

Indication(s)= _____

Side Effects= _____

Types/ Examples= _____

Transdermal Patch:

MOA = _____

Indication(s)=_____

Side Effects=_____

Types/ Examples=_____

Combined Oral Contraception:

MOA = _____

Indication(s)=_____

Side Effects=_____

Types/ Examples=_____

Progesterone Only Pill:

MOA = _____

Indication(s)=_____

Side Effects=_____

Types/ Examples=_____

Emergency Contraception:

MOA = _____

Indication(s)=_____

Side Effects=_____

Types/ Examples=_____

Breast Disorders

Mastitis: S. aureus

Sx: Unilateral breast pain, tenderness, warmth, swelling

PE: Cracked nipples and fissures

Dx:

_____   Tx:

_____

_____

Breast Abscess: S. aureus

Sx: Red, mass, pain, fluctuance, induration

PE:

Dx:

_____   Tx:

_____

_____

Fibrocystic Breast Changes: Typically presents prior to menstruation

Sx:

PE:

Dx:

_____   Tx:

_____

_____

Fibroadenoma: **Common benign solid tumor**

Sx: Round, firm, discrete, mobile, non-tender mass

PE:

Dx:

_____

_____

_____

Tx:

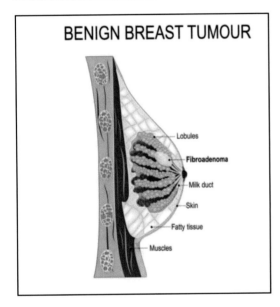

BENIGN BREAST TUMOUR

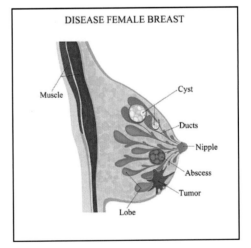

DISEASE FEMALE BREAST

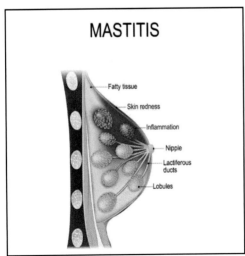

MASTITIS

Breast Cancer

Invasive Ductal Carcinoma:

Sx: Can be asymptomatic

PE:

Dx: Mammogram

_____

_____

_____

Tx:

Invasive ductal carcinoma

Invasive Lobular Carcinoma: Most common type

Sx: Can be asymptomatic

PE:

Dx: Mammogram

_____

_____

_____

Tx:

Paget's Disease of the Breast:

Sx: Itchy, scaling rash on the nipples & areola

PE:

Dx:

_____

_____

_____

Tx:

Breast Cancer Screening and Prevention:

Other GYN Dysplasias & Carcinomas

Cervical Dysplasia:

Sx:

PE:

Dx: Pap smear
  ASC - US
  LSIL - low grade (CIN I)
  ASC - H
  HSIL - high grade (CIN II, III)

_____   Tx:

_____

_____

Cervical Cancer:

Risk Factors: Human papilloma virus (HPV) *in Infectious Disease*, smoking

Sx: Post-coital bleeding or spotting

PE:

Dx: Pap smear
  ASC - US
  LSIL
  HSIL

_____   Tx:

_____

_____

Cervical Cancer Screening:

HPV vaccination:

Endometrial Hyperplasia:

Risk Factors: Prolonged unopposed estrogen, chronic anovulation, obesity, PCOS, Tamoxifen use

Sx: Abnormal uterine bleeding

PE:

Dx:

_____

_____

_____

Tx:

Endometrial Cancer: **Most common GYN malignancy**

Risk Factors: Endometrial hyperplasia, high estrogen exposure, obesity, PCOS

Sx: Postmenopausal bleeding

PE:

Dx:

_____

_____   Tx:

_____

Ovarian Cancer: **Epithelial carcinoma is most common**

Risk Factors: Nulligravida, early menarche, late menopause, endometriosis

Early Sx:

Late Sx:

PE: Adnexal mass, abdominal bloating

Dx:

_____   Tx:

_____

_____

Protective Factors: OCP use, breastfeeding

Vaginal Cancer: **RARE**

Risk Factors: Smoking, HPV, multiple partners, Diethylstilbestrol (DES)

Sx: Postmenopausal & postcoital bleeding

PE: Vaginal mass

Dx:

_____   Tx:

_____

_____

Vulvar Cancer:

Sx: Vaginal pruritus

PE: Red, white ulcerative, or raised crusted lesion

Dx:

_____

_____

_____

Tx:

Postmenopausal Bleeding:

Sx: Vaginal bleeding occurring after menopause

PE:

Dx:

_____   Tx:

_____

_____

Female Reproductive Organ Concerns

Polycystic Ovarian Syndrome (PCOS):

Sx: Amenorrhea, obesity, hirsutism, polycystic ovaries, increased LH & FSH, androgen excess

PE:

Dx:

_____   Tx:

_____

_____

Ovarian Cyst: **Most common are follicular cyst**

Sx: Pelvic pain, bloating

PE: Palpable abdominal mass

Dx:

_____   Tx:

_____

_____

Ovarian Cyst Rupture:

Sx: Sudden abdominal pain, fever, vomiting

PE:

Dx:

_____   Tx:

_____

_____

Ovarian Torsion: EMERGENCY!!!

Sx: Waxing and waning pain, N/V/D, sudden, sharp, unilateral pain

PE:

Dx: Transvaginal US

_____   Tx:

_____

_____

Endometriosis:

Sx: Dyspareunia, dyschezia, dysmenorrhea

PE: Uterus is fixed and retroflexed

Dx:

_____

_____

_____

Tx:

ENDOMETRIOSIS

Chronic Endometriosis:

Sx: Abdominal swelling, abnormal vaginal bleeding

PE:

Dx:

_____

_____   Tx:

_____

Leiomyoma: Uterine fibroids

Sx:

PE:

Dx: US and/or MRI

_____

_____

_____

Tx:

Uterine fibroids

Adenomyoma:

Sx: Cramping, metrorrhagia, dysmenorrhea

PE:

Dx:

_____   **Tx:**

_____

_____

Bartholin Cyst & Abscess:

Sx: Vulvar pain and/or mass

PE:

Dx:

_____   **Tx:**

_____

_____

Toxic Shock Syndrome:

Sx: Rapid onset fever, body aches, headache, chills

PE:

Dx:

_____   **Tx:**

_____

_____

Misc. Women's Health

Bladder Prolapse (Cystocele): Anterior vagina

Sx: Vaginal fullness "heaviness", urinary urgency & frequency

PE:

Dx:

_____   Tx:

_____

_____

Rectal Prolapse (Rectocele): Posterior wall

Sx:

PE:

Dx:

_____   Tx:

_____

_____

Uterine Prolapse: Uterine herniation into the vagina

Sx: Vaginal protrusion & pressure

PE:

Dx:

_____

_____

_____

Tx:

Types of Pelvic Organ Prolapse

Normal Anatomy   Rectocele

Cystocele   Uterine prolapse

Uncomplicated Pregnancy

Hormones

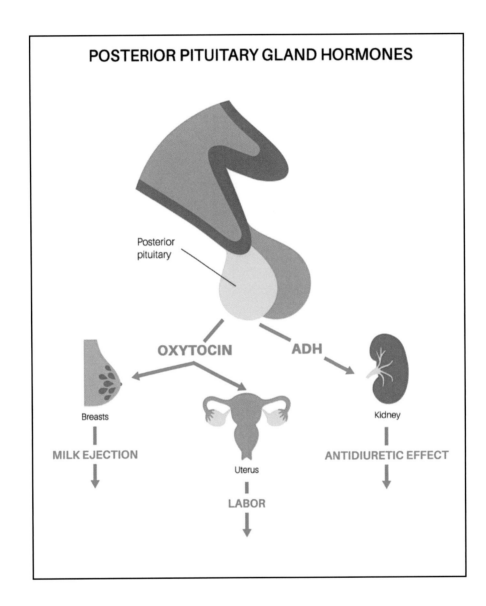

Trimesters

1st Trimester: Weeks 1-12

Fetal heart tones by 12 weeks

Chronic villus sampling 10-12 weeks

2nd Trimester: Weeks 13-27

15-18 weeks = amniocentesis

24 weeks = 1 hour glucose challenge test

3rd Trimester: Weeks 28-40

28-30 weeks = Rhogam injection if Rh negative

35-37 = group B strep

36-40 = gonorrhea & chlamydia cultures

UA & blood glucose

Pregnancy Terms:

Hegar's sign = softening of the uterus, possible early sign of pregnancy

Goodell's sign = softening of the cervix, possible early sign of pregnancy

Chadwick's sign = increased vascularity, purplish-blue color. Possible early sign of pregnancy

Naegele's rule = 1st day of last menses + 7 days - 3 months + 1 year

Gravida: Number of times a woman has been pregnant

Parity: Number of pregnancies that led to a birth either at or after 20 weeks

T (term) = number born at 37 weeks or older

P (preterm) = born after 20 weeks but before 37 weeks

A (abortion) = all pregnancy losses prior to 20 weeks

L (living) = infant who lives beyond 30 days

Nulligravida: Woman who currently is not pregnant and never has been pregnant

Primigravida: Woman who currently is pregnant and has never been pregnant before

Multigravida: Woman who currently is pregnant and who has been pregnant before

Nullipara: Woman who has never completed a pregnancy beyond 20 weeks

Primipara: Woman who has delivered a fetus or fetuses born alive or dead with an estimate length of gestation of 20 weeks for the first time

Multipara: Woman who has delivered a fetus or fetuses born alive or dead with an estimate length of gestation of 20 weeks multiple times

Women's Health Tidbits:

Pregnancy is a hypercoagulable state

Appendectomy is the most common surgery during pregnancy

The placenta secretes estrogen, progesterone, relaxin, and hCG

Vaginal pH during pregnancy = 3.5-6.0

Pregnancy increases cardiac output, decreases blood pressure, and increases total red blood cells

Decreased hematocrit = physiologic anemia

Fundal Height:

       12 weeks - above pubic symphysis

       16 weeks - midway between pubis & umbilicus

       20 weeks - umbilicus

       38 weeks - 2-3 cm below xiphoid

Vaccines in Pregnancy:

Inactivated influenza can be given in 3rd trimester during flu season

Cannot give live attenuated vaccines (MMR, varicella)

Tdap encouraged in pregnancy, no harm to fetus, between 27 & 36 weeks

Stages of Labor

Apgar Score

Intrapartum

Pregnancy Complications

Ectopic Pregnancy: Pregnancy outside uterine cavity - most commonly occurs in the fallopian tube

Sx: Unilateral pelvic pain, vaginal bleeding, referred shoulder or upper abdominal pain

PE:

Dx: B-hCG > 1500

　　US "ring of fire"

_____　　Tx:

_____

_____

Gestational Trophoblastic Disease: Molar pregnancy - Choriocarcinoma

Sx: Painless vaginal bleeding

PE:

Dx: hCG higher than expected

　　US = "snow storm" "swiss cheese"

_____

_____

_____

Tx:

Complete =

Incomplete =

Spontaneous Abortion = before 20 weeks
Threatened: Vaginal bleeding, closed cervix

Sx:

_____   Tx:

_____

_____

Incomplete: Cervical os dilated with some products of conception visible < 20 weeks

Sx:

_____   Tx:

_____

_____

Inevitable: Cervical os dilated without products < 20 weeks

Sx:

_____   Tx:

_____

_____

Missed Abortion: Death of fetus without symptons < 20 weeks

Sx:

_____   Tx:

_____

_____

Dx: US

Elective Abortion:

Sx:

PE:

Dx:

_____   Tx:

_____

_____

Infertility:

Sx:

PE:

Dx: Hysterosalpingogram, semen analysis

_____   Tx:

_____

_____

Multiple Gestation:

Dizygotic (fraternal): Fertilization of 2 ova by 2 different sperm

Monozygotic (identical): Fertilization of 1 ovum that splits

Sx:

PE:

Dx:

_____   Tx:

_____

_____

Incompetent Cervix: **Premature cervical shortening or dilation in the second or early third trimesters**

Sx:

PE: Cervical dilation > 2 cm, painless

Dx:

_____   Tx:

_____

_____

Rh Factor: **Babies at risk = (-Rh) mother, (+Rh) father or unknown**

1st pregnancy is good, 2nd at risk

Sx:

PE:

Dx:

_____   Tx:

_____

_____

Preeclampsia:

Sx: Hypertension, proteinuria +/- edema after 20 weeks

Dx: Mild: 140/90 - 160/110 & proteinuria > 300 mg/24 hour or +1 dipstick

Dx: Severe: > 160/110 & proteinuria > 5g/24 hour or +3 on dipstick

Tx:

_____

_____

_____

HELLP (Hemolysis, Elevated Liver Enzymes, and Low Platelets):

Sx: Abdominal pain, vision changes

PE:

Dx:

Tx:

_____

_____

_____

Eclampsia: Hypertension + proteinuria + seizures or coma

Sx:

PE:

Dx: Same as Preeclampsia

Tx:

_____

_____

_____

Gestational Hypertension: **Symptoms after 20 weeks & resolves by 12 weeks postpartum**

Sx:

PE:

Dx: BP > 150/90

_____   **Tx:**

_____

_____

Chronic Hypertension: **Symptoms before 20 weeks**

Sx:

PE:

Dx: Mild: 140/90

　　Moderate: 150/100

　　Severe: 160/110

_____   **Tx:**

_____

_____

Uterine Rupture:

Sx: Excessive vaginal bleeding, pain between contractions

PE:

Dx:

_____   **Tx:**

_____

_____

Gestational Diabetes:

Sx:

PE:

Dx:

Test 1: 1 hour, 50g, glucose challenge test (performed between 24-28 weeks)

Test 2: If 1 hour test failed, proceed to 3 hour, 100g, glucose tolerance test.
    To fail the 3 hour test there must be 2 abnormal values
    Initial fasting: 95
    1st hour: 180
    2nd hour: 155
    3rd hour: 140

_____   **Tx:**

_____

_____

Pregestational Diabetes:

Sx:

PE:

Dx: Fasting blood glucose > 126, A1C > 6.5, random blood glucose > 200

_____   **Tx:**

_____

_____

Preterm Labor: **Labor before 37 weeks**

Sx: Contractions, back ache

PE:

Dx:

_____   **Tx:**

_____

_____

Placental Abruption: Separation of the placenta partially or totally from its implantation site before delivery

Risk Factors: Smoking, cocaine, trauma

Sx: Bleeding, abdominal PAIN

PE:

Dx: US

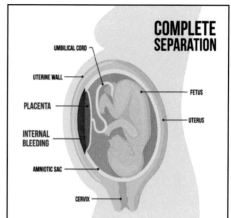

_____

_____

_____

Tx:

Placenta Previa: Placenta that is implanted either over or near the internal cervical os

Risk Factors: Prior C-section, multiple gestation, multiple induced abortions

Sx: PAINLESS vaginal bleeding

PE:

Dx:

_____   Tx:

_____

_____

<u>Classifications:</u>

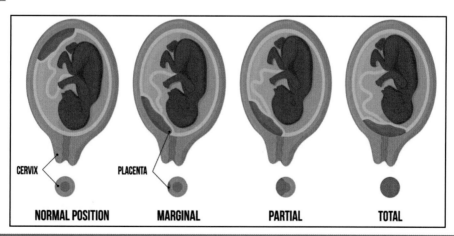

Labor & Delivery Complications

Premature Rupture Of Membranes (PROM): **Rupture of amniotic sac before regular contractions start.**

Preterm PROM (PROM): PROM before 37 weeks gestation

Risk Factors:

Sx:

PE:

Dx: Nitrazine paper test: Turns blue if pH >7, "ferning" on microscopy

_____   **Tx:**

_____

_____

Placental Insufficiency: Placenta is damaged or doesn't develop appropriately

Sx:

PE:

Dx:

_____   **Tx:**

_____

_____

Umbilical Cord Prolapse: Umbilical cord protrudes out of vagina

Sx:

PE: Bradycardia, variable decelerations

Dx:

_____

_____

_____

Tx:

Breech: **Presenting with buttocks and/or feet at cervix**

Sx:

PE:

Dx:

_____   Tx:

_____

_____

Types:

Complete breech   Frank breech   Incomplete breech

Shoulder Dystocia:

Causes: Small pelvis, big baby, female mutilation or tumor, narrow vaginal canal

Sx:

PE:

Dx: Turtle sign

_____   Tx:

_____

_____

Categories: 1. Problem of power - uterine contractions

2. Problem of passenger - macrosomia, position

3. Problem of passage - uterus or soft tissue abnormalities

Postpartum Hemorrhage: 4Ts: Tone, trauma, tissue (retained placental tissue), thrombin

Most common cause is UTERINE ATONY

Uterine atony:

Genital tract trauma:

Retained placental tissue:

Coagulation disorders:

Sx:

PE: Loss of > 500 mL within 24 hours after vaginal delivery

> 1000mL after C-section

Dx:

_____   Tx:

_____

_____

Sheehan Syndrome:

Causes: Hemorrhage, hypotension, shock

Sx:

PE:

Dx:

_____   Tx:

_____

_____

Cesarean Section: Surgical procedure to deliver baby/babies through the abdominal wall

_____   Tx:

_____

_____

Endometritis: Inflammation of endometrium (most common infection after childbirth)

Risk Factors: C-section, PROM, vaginal delivery, D&C

Sx: Fever, tachycardia, foul smell

PE:

Dx:

_____   Tx:

_____

_____

Perineal Lacerations: Tearing of perineum during childbirth

Sx:

PE: Depends on the degree of the tear/laceration

Dx:

_____   Tx:

_____

_____

Puerperium or Postpartum Period: Lasts 6 weeks

- **Placental implant site shrinks by ½ after delivery**
- **Lochia rubra: Normal postpartum discharge, blood, tissue, & decidua - stops after 5 or 6 weeks**
- **No vigorous exercise for 6-7 weeks**
- **Cervix shinks to 1 cm by the end of 1st week**
- **Vagina returns to antepartum condition by 3rd week**
- **Pelvic floor muscles return to original position, but are pre-disposed to cystocele, & rectocele**
- **Bladder capacity returns to normal by 6 weeks**
- **Ovulation can happen as early as 27 days after birth or 6 months if breastfeeding**
  - o **Ovulation is suppressed by increased prolactin**

Postpartum Depression:

Sx: Depressive symptoms that can start during pregnancy and last up to 12 months

PE:

Dx:

_____   **Tx:**

_____

_____

*Anorexia: **In Psych***

*Vaginal Diseases/Infections: **In ID***

*Premenstrual Dysphoric Disorder (PMDD): **In Psych***

Medications

_____: MOA = _____

Indication(s)=_____

Side Effects = _____

Types/ Examples = _____

_____

_____

_____: MOA = _____

Indication(s)=_____

Side Effects = _____

Types/ Examples = _____

_____

_____

_____: MOA = _____

Indication(s)=_____

Side Effects = _____

Types/ Examples = _____

_____

_____

_____: MOA = _____

Indication(s)=_____

Side Effects = _____

Types/ Examples = _____

_____

_____

_____: MOA = _____

Indication(s)=_____

Side Effects = _____

Types/ Examples = _____

_____

Medications

_____: MOA = _____

Indication(s)=_____

Side Effects = _____

Types/ Examples = _____

_____

_____

_____: MOA = _____

Indication(s)=_____

Side Effects = _____

Types/ Examples = _____

_____

_____

_____: MOA = _____

Indication(s)=_____

Side Effects = _____

Types/ Examples = _____

_____

_____

_____: MOA = _____

Indication(s)=_____

Side Effects = _____

Types/ Examples = _____

_____

_____

_____: MOA = _____

Indication(s)=_____

Side Effects = _____

Types/ Examples = _____

_____

Neurology

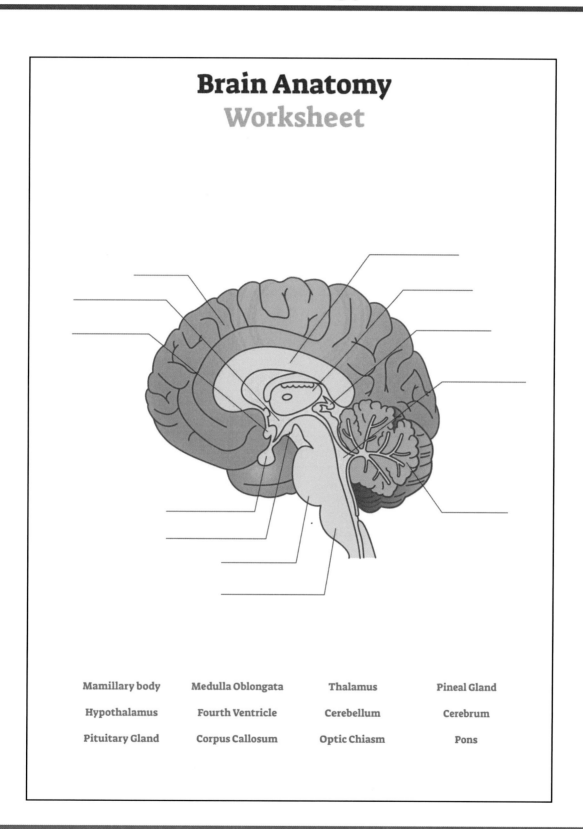

Brain Anatomy
Worksheet

Mamillary body	Medulla Oblongata	Thalamus	Pineal Gland
Hypothalamus	Fourth Ventricle	Cerebellum	Cerebrum
Pituitary Gland	Corpus Callosum	Optic Chiasm	Pons

Peripheral Nerve Disorders

Complex Regional Pain Syndrome: Chronic pain in a specific body region
Most common = extremities

Sx: Pain, swelling, skin changes, vasomotor instability

PE:

Dx:

_____   Tx:

_____

_____

Guillain-Barré Syndrome: Associated with campylobacter jejuni

Sx:

PE:

Dx: LP with increased CSF protein
    Check vital capacity for lung function

_____

_____

_____

Tx:

Peripheral Neuropathy:

Sx: Loss of sensation, paresthesia of extremities

PE:

Dx: EMG

_____   Tx:

_____

_____

Diabetic Neuropathy: **Often associated with poor glycemic control**

Sx:

PE:

Dx: EMG

_____   Tx:

_____

_____

Bell's Palsy: **CN VII - associated with HSV (prodrome viral illness)**

Sx:

PE: Paralysis of CN VII distribution, unable to lift eyebrow

Dx:

_____

_____

_____

Tx:

Trigeminal Neuralgia: **Demyelination & compression of CN V**

Sx: Intermittent zapping facial pain along CN V distribution

PE:

Dx:

TRIGEMINAL NEURALGIA

V1 Ophthalmic nerve

V2 Maxillary nerve

Mandibular nerve V3

Cervical nerve

_____

_____

_____

Tx:

Movement Disorders

Essential Tremor: Autosomal dominant - worse with caffeine, better with alcohol

Sx:

PE:

Dx: Clinical

_____   Tx:

_____

_____

Huntington's Disease: Autosomal dominant

Sx:

PE:

Dx: MRI = atrophy of basal ganglia

_____   Tx:

_____

_____

Parkinson's Disease: Low dopamine from substantia nigra

Sx:

PE: Pill rolling, cogwheel rigidity, bradykinesia, shuffling gait, masked faces

Dx:

_____

_____

_____

Tx:

Infectious Neurologic Disorders

Encephalitis: Viral infection of brain tissue

Sx: Altered mental status, headache, seizures

PE:

Dx: Lumbar puncture

_____   Tx:

_____

_____

Bacterial Meningitis:

Sx:

PE: + Kernig, + Brudzinski

Dx: LP = high protein, low glucose, high pressure

_____   Tx:

_____

_____

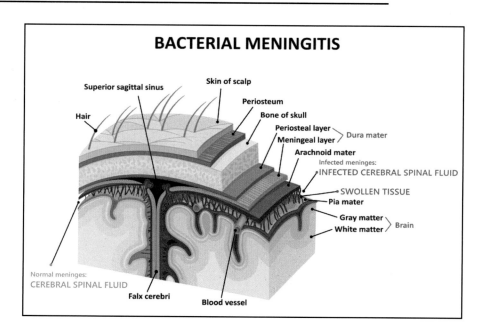

BACTERIAL MENINGITIS

Superior sagittal sinus
Skin of scalp
Hair
Periosteum
Bone of skull
Periosteal layer
Meningeal layer
Dura mater
Arachnoid mater
Infected meninges:
INFECTED CEREBRAL SPINAL FLUID
SWOLLEN TISSUE
Pia mater
Gray matter
White matter
Brain
Normal meninges:
CEREBRAL SPINAL FLUID
Falx cerebri
Blood vessel

Viral Meningitis:

Sx:

PE:

Dx: LP + WBC, normal pressure & glucose

_____   **Tx:**

_____

_____

Brain Abscess:

Sx: Headache, altered mental status, fever

PE:

Dx:

_____   **Tx:**

_____

_____

Spine Disorders

Spinal Cord Compression: Trauma

Sx: Loss of motor/sensory reflexes depending on level of trauma to spinal cord

PE:

Dx:

_____   Tx:

_____

_____

Brown-Séquard Syndrome: Traumatic hemisection of spinal cord

Sx: Ipsilateral loss vibration/proprioception - contralateral loss of pain/temp

PE:

Dx: MRI

_____   Tx:

_____

_____

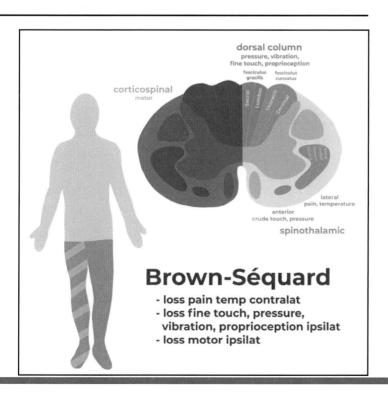

Neurocognitive & Neuromuscular Disorders

Delirium: Rapid onset, short-term, reversible

Sx: Acute, fluctuating change in mental status

PE:

Dx:

_____   Tx:

_____

_____

Dementia: Gradual, irreversible memory loss

    Alzheimer's: Most common cause

        Sx:

        Dx:

        _____   Tx:

        _____

    Lewy Body: Parkinson's

        Sx:

        Dx:

        _____   Tx:

        _____

    Frontotemporal: Personality/language changes (younger patients)

        Sx:

        Dx:

        _____   Tx:

        _____

    Vascular: Correlated with cardiovascular disease

        Sx:

        Dx:

        _____   Tx:

        _____

Mild Cognitive Impairment: **No effect on ADLs**

Sx:

PE:

Dx: Montreal Cognitive Assessment (MoCa)

_____   Tx:

_____

_____

Cerebral Palsy: **Trauma - hypoxia at birth**

Sx:

PE:

Dx: MRI of the brain

_____   Tx:

_____

_____

Multiple Sclerosis: **Autoimmune**

Sx:

PE: Optic neuritis (Marcus-Gunn pupil)

Dx: LP = oligoclonal bands, MRI of spine

_____   Tx:

_____

_____

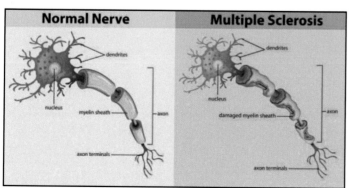

Myasthenia Gravis: **Autoimmune**

Sx: Muscles weaken and fatigue = hallmark of the disease: ptosis, diplopia

PE:

Dx: Ice bag test

_____   **Tx:**

_____

_____

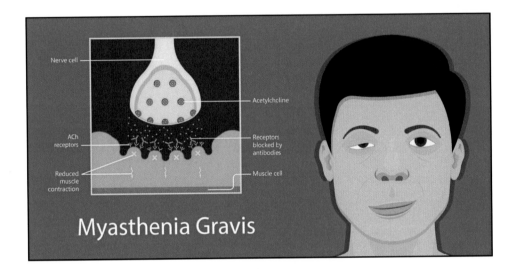

Emergent, Vascular, & Associated Neuro Disorders

Intracerebral Hemorrhage: Intraparenchymal bleeding

Sx:

PE:

Dx: Non-contrast head CT

_____   Tx:

_____

_____

Epidural Hematoma: Arterial (middle meningeal artery)

Sx:

PE:

Dx: CT with biconvex lens

_____   Tx:

_____

_____

Subdural Hematoma: Blood below dura (venous bridging veins)

Sx:

PE:

Dx: CT with crescent

_____   Tx:

_____

_____

EPIDURAL HEMATOMA VS SUBDURAL HEMATOMA

Subarachnoid Hemorrhage: **Ruptured aneurysm**

Sx: Thunderclap headache "worst headache of their life"

PE:

Dx: LP with xanthochromia

_____

_____

_____

Tx:

Subarachnoid hemorrhage

Aneurysm

Arachnoid

The aneurysm formed between the arteries ruptures.
Bleeding occurs in the subarachnoid space, causing various disorders.

Cerebral Aneurysm: **Weak, bulging spot of artery (AICA, PICA, MCA)**

Sx:

PE:

Dx: CTA

_____   Tx:

_____

_____

Hydrocephalus: Accumulation of cerebral spinal fluid
Communicating:
Non-communicating:

Sx:

PE:

Dx: CT/MRI, US in infants

_____   Tx:

_____

_____

MRI scan ventricles from top view

Normal ventricles

Enlarged ventricles

Normal ventricles

Hydrocephalus (Enlarged ventricles)

Normal Pressure Hydrocephalus: Enlarged ventricles with normal pressure

Sx: "Wacky, wobbly, wet"

PE:

Dx:

_____   Tx:

_____

_____

Idiopathic Intracranial Hypertension: High intracranial pressure

Sx:

PE:

Dx: LP with high opening pressure

_____   Tx:

_____

_____

Ischemic Stroke:

Sx:

PE:

Dx: Non-contrast head CT

_____   Tx:

_____

_____

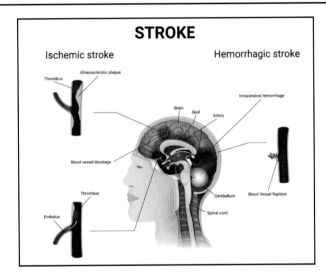

Vertebral **(vertigo)**

Basilar **(coma, CN palsy) – also affects PICA, AICA**

ACA **(leg weak, urinary incontinence)**

MCA **(face/arm weak, aphasia)**

PCA **(vision)**

Transient Ischemic Attack (TIA): Focal neural deficits that resolve within 1 hour

Sx:

PE:

Dx: Non-contrast head CT

_____   Tx:

_____

_____

Syncope: **Loss of consciousness**

Sx:

PE:

Dx:

_____   Tx:

_____

_____

Pituitary Apoplexy: **Infarct or hemorrhage of pituitary gland**

Sx:

PE:

Dx: CT/MRI

_____   Tx:

_____

_____

Skull Fractures:

Sx:

PE: Battle sign, racoon eyes

Dx: CT

_____   Tx:

_____

_____

Concussion:

Sx:

PE:

Dx: Glasgow Coma Scale

_____

_____ | **Glasgow Coma Scale** |

_____

Tx:

Postconcussive Syndrome:

Sx: Headache, memory difficulties, fatigue

PE:

Dx:

_____   Tx:

_____

_____

Traumatic Brain Injury (TBI):

Sx:

PE:

Dx: Serial Glasgow Coma Scale, non-contrast head CT

_____   Tx:

_____

_____

Wernicke Encephalopathy: Thiamine deficiency associated with EtOH

Sx: Ataxia, confusion, nystagmus

PE:

Dx: MRI = punctate hemorrhages

_____   Tx:

_____

_____

VP Shunt Malformation: Can lead to hydrocephalus

Sx:

PE:

Dx:

_____   Tx:

_____

_____

Headaches

Cluster Headache: **Unilateral**

Sx: Ice pick headache lasting 15 minutes to 3 hours

PE:

Dx:

_____

_____

_____

Tx:

Migraine Headaches: **Unilateral**

Sx: Throbbing pain, nausea, photophobia, +/- aura

PE:

Dx:

_____

_____

_____

Tx:

Tension Headaches: **Bilateral**

Sx: Band-like pain around head

PE:

Dx:

_____

_____

_____

Tx:

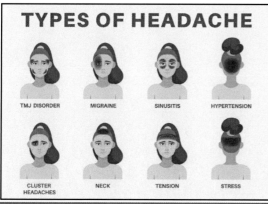

TYPES OF HEADACHE

TMJ DISORDER   MIGRAINE   SINUSITIS   HYPERTENSION

CLUSTER HEADACHES   NECK   TENSION   STRESS

Congenital Neurologic Disorders

Chiari Malformation

Sx: Headache, imbalance, hydrocephalus

PE:

Dx: MRI

_____

_____

_____

Seizure Disorders

Partial Seizure: Focal

Simple: No loss of consciousness

Complex: Loss of consciousness

Sx:

PE:

Dx: EEG

_____   Tx:

_____

_____

Generalized Seizures: **Midbrain or brainstem**

    Tonic-colonic (grand mal) = rigid & convulsions

        Sx:

        PE:

        Dx:

        _____   Tx:

        _____

    Absence (petite mal) = loss of consciousness without convulsions

        Sx:

        PE:

        Dx:

        _____   Tx:

        _____

    Myoclonus = twitching, no loss of consciousness

        Sx:

        PE:

        Dx:

        _____   Tx:

        _____

Status Epilepticus: 5+ minutes of continuous seizures or 2+ separate seizures where there is not a recovery of consciousness

Sx:

PE:

Dx: Always check blood glucose

_____   Tx:

_____

_____

Febrile Seizures: Convulsions with high temp > 38 °C

Sx:

PE:

Dx:

_____   Tx:

_____

_____

Epilepsy: 2+ seizures, chronic, usually starts in childhood

Sx:

PE:

Dx:

_____   Tx:

_____

_____

Misc. Neuro Concerns

Subclavian Steal Syndrome: Retrograde blood flow down ipsilateral vertebral artery

Sx: Hearing loss, tinnitus, changes in vision, vertigo, ataxia, syncope

PE:

Dx:

_____   Tx:

_____

_____

Hemangioma: Benign vascular malformation

Sx:

PE:

Dx: Doppler US, MRI, or CT of hemangioma

_____   Tx:

_____

_____

Glioblastoma: Aggressive form of brain cancer

Sx:

PE:

Dx: Brain MRI

_____   Tx:

_____

_____

*Giant Cell (Temporal) Arteritis: **In Cardio***

*Cauda Equina Syndrome: **In MSK***

*Spinal Epidural Abscess: **In MSK***

*Arteriovenous Malformation: **In Cardiac***

*Tourette Syndrome: **In Psych***

Medications

_____: MOA = _____

Indication(s)=_____

Side Effects = _____

Types/ Examples = _____

_____

_____

_____: MOA = _____

Indication(s)=_____

Side Effects = _____

Types/ Examples = _____

_____

_____

_____: MOA = _____

Indication(s)=_____

Side Effects = _____

Types/ Examples = _____

_____

_____

_____: MOA = _____

Indication(s)=_____

Side Effects = _____

Types/ Examples = _____

_____

_____

_____: MOA = _____

Indication(s)=_____

Side Effects = _____

Types/ Examples = _____

_____

Medications

_____ : MOA = _____

Indication(s)=_____

Side Effects = _____

Types/ Examples = _____

_____

_____

_____ : MOA = _____

Indication(s)=_____

Side Effects = _____

Types/ Examples = _____

_____

_____

_____ : MOA = _____

Indication(s)=_____

Side Effects = _____

Types/ Examples = _____

_____

_____

_____ : MOA = _____

Indication(s)=_____

Side Effects = _____

Types/ Examples = _____

_____

_____

_____ : MOA = _____

Indication(s)=_____

Side Effects = _____

Types/ Examples = _____

_____

Hematology

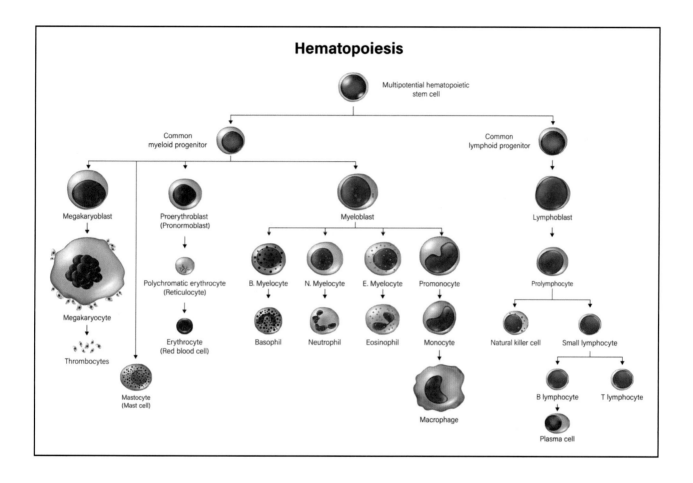

Hematopoiesis

Multipotential hematopoietic stem cell

Common myeloid progenitor

Common lymphoid progenitor

Megakaryoblast

Proerythroblast (Pronormoblast)

Myeloblast

Lymphoblast

Megakaryocyte

Polychromatic erythrocyte (Reticulocyte)

B. Myelocyte

N. Myelocyte

E. Myelocyte

Promonocyte

Prolymphocyte

Thrombocytes

Erythrocyte (Red blood cell)

Basophil

Neutrophil

Eosinophil

Monocyte

Natural killer cell

Small lymphocyte

Mastocyte (Mast cell)

Macrophage

B lymphocyte

T lymphocyte

Plasma cell

Anemias
Microcytic = low MCV < 80 fL

Iron Deficiency Anemia:

Sx:

PE: Fatigue, koilonychias, angular cheilitis

Dx:

_____   **Tx:**

_____

_____

Thalassemia:

Alpha-Thalassemia: 4

Sx:

Dx: Hemoglobin, RBC, peripheral smear

Beta-Thalassemia: 2

Sx:

Dx: Same as above

_____   **Tx:**

_____

_____

Alpha-Thalassemia	Beta-Thalassemia

Macrocytic: High MCV > 100 fL

Vitamin B12 Deficiency:

Causes: Veganism, pernicious anemia, bypass surgery

Sx: Glossitis, neuro symptoms

PE:

Dx: Labs = high MMA, high homocysteine

_____   Tx:

_____

_____

Pernicious Anemia: Can't absorb B12

Sx:

PE:

Dx: + shilling test, CBC

_____   Tx:

_____

_____

Folate Deficiency:

Causes: Alcoholism, pregnancy

Sx:

PE: Glossitis, neuro symptoms less common

Dx:

_____   Tx:

_____

_____

Myelodysplastic Syndrome: Precancerous - can lead to AML

Sx:

PE: Labs = pancytopenia

Dx:

_____

_____

_____

Tx:

Normocytic: Normal MCV 80 - 100 fL

Aplastic Anemia:

Sx:

PE: Petechiae, ecchymosis, weakness, pallor

Dx: Bone marrow biopsy

_____

_____

_____

Tx:

APLASTIC ANEMIA

Platelets

Red blood cells

Bone marrow

White blood cells

Anemia of Chronic Disease: Micro - or normocytic anemia

Sx:

PE:

Dx: Low Fe, low TIBC, high ferritin

_____   Tx:

_____

_____

Hemolytic Anemia:

Sx: Fatigue, jaundice

PE:

Dx: CBC, unconjugated (indirect) biliruben

_____   Tx:

_____

_____

Autoimmune:

Causes: Idiopathic, CLL, autoimmune (SLE, RA, etc.)

Sx:

PE:

Dx: + Coombs

_____   **Tx:**

_____

_____

Cold Ab Hemolytic Anemia:

Sx:

PE:

Dx: + Coombs

_____   **Tx:**

_____

_____

Hereditary Spherocytosis: Red blood cells destroyed in spleen

Sx:

PE:

Dx: + Osmotic fragility, - Coombs

_____

_____

_____

Hemolysis

Normal red blood cell (erythrocyte)

Spherocyte (erythrocytes that are sphere-shaped)

Rupturing of erythrocyte, and the release of contents into blood plasma

Tx:

Paroxysmal Nocturnal Hemoglobinuria (PNH): Idiopathic

Sx: Dark urine in the morning

PE:

Dx:

_____   Tx:

_____

_____

G6PD Deficiency: X-linked recessive, patients with ancestry from Africa, Europe, and Asia

Sx:

PE:

Dx: + Heinz bodies & bite cells, - Coombs

_____   Tx:

_____

_____

Sickle Cell Disease (Anemia): Autosomal recessive

Sx: Pain crisis, acute chest syndrome

PE:

Dx: Howell-Jolly bodies, high reticulocyte count

ANEMIA

Sickle cell

Normal red blood cell

Abnormal hemoglobin

Normal hemoglobin

Sickle cells blocking blood flow

_____

_____

_____

Tx:

Hematologic Malignancies

Hodgkin Lymphoma: Bimodal age distribution, associated with EBV

Sx:

PE:

Dx: Lymph node biopsy = Reed-Sternberg cells

_____   **Tx:**

_____

_____

Non-Hodgkin Lymphoma: Most common in patients > 50 years of age and with HIV, worse prognosis

Sx:

PE:

Dx: Lymph node biopsy = Reed-Sternberg cells

_____

_____

_____

Tx:

Acute Lymphocytic Leukemia (ALL): **Seen in kids**

Sx: Fever, bone pain, bruising, fatigue

PE:

Dx: CBC with differential, peripheral blood smear

_____   **Tx:**

_____

_____

Acute Myeloid Leukemia (AML): **Immature myeloid cell proliferation**

Sx: Gingival hyperplasia

PE:

Dx: Bone marrow biopsy = Auer rods

_____   **Tx:**

_____

_____

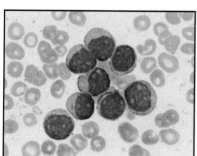

Chronic Lymphocytic Leukemia (CLL):

Sx:

PE:

Dx: High WBC, smudge cells

_____   Tx:

_____

_____

Chronic Myeloid Leukemia (CML): **Seen in adults**

Sx:

PE:

Dx: Philadelphia chromosome

_____   Tx:

_____

_____

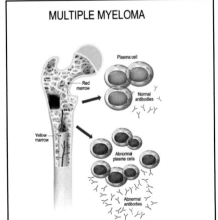

Multiple Myeloma (MM): **Malignancy of plasma cells**

Sx:

PE: UA - Bence Jones proteins
    X-ray - lytic lesions

Dx:

_____

_____

_____

Tx:

Clotting Pathway

von Willebrand Factor

Hypercoagulability Disorders

Protein C & S Deficiencies:

Complications: Pulmonary embolism & deep vein thrombosis

Sx:

PE:

Dx:

_____   **Tx:**

_____

_____

Factor V Leiden:

Complications: Pulmonary embolism & deep vein thrombosis

Sx:

PE:

Dx: CBC, other blood tests

_____   **Tx:**

_____

_____

Thrombocytopenias

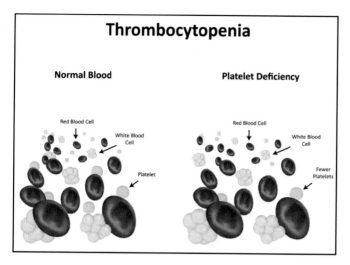

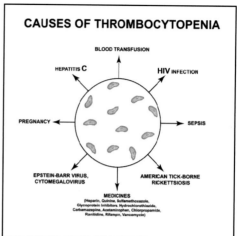

Idiopathic Thrombocytopenia Purpura (ITP): **Autoimmune**

Sx:

PE:

Dx: Low platelets, normal PT & PTT, + Coombs

Tx:

_____

_____

_____

Thrombotic Thrombocytopenia Purpura (TTP): **ADAMTS13**

Sx:

PE:

Dx: Pentad = thrombocytopenia, hemolytic anemia, renal failure, fever, neuro symptoms

Tx:

_____

_____

_____

Hemolytic Uremic Syndrome (HUS): **E. coli infection**

Sx:

PE:

Dx: Triad = thrombocytopenia, hemolytic anemia, renal failure

Tx:

_____

_____

_____

Disseminated Intravascular Coagulation (DIC): **Simultaneous clot formation & breakdown**

Sx: Thrombosis, excessive bleeding

PE:

Dx:

Tx:

_____

_____

_____

Heparin-Induced Thrombocytopenia (HIT):

Sx:

PE:

Dx: Increased bleeding time, normal PT & PTT

Tx:

_____

_____

_____

Bleeding Disorders

Hemophilia A (VIII) & B (IV-Christmas): X-linked recessive

Sx:

PE:

Dx: Factor assay, long PTT

_____

_____

_____

Tx:

Hemophilia C (XI): Autosomal recessive - more common in patients of Ashkenazi Jewish ancestry

Sx:

PE:

Dx: Prolonged PTT

_____   Tx:

_____

_____

Von Willebrand Disease (vWB): Autosomal dominant - more common in women

Sx:

PE:

Dx: Low vWB, long bleeding time, long PTT

_____   Tx:

_____

_____

Myeloproliferative Disorders

Primary Polycythemia Vera: Marrow malignancy with RBC overproduction

Sx: Pruritis after shower

PE:

Dx: JAK2 mutation, high hemoglobin & hematocrit

_____   Tx:

_____

_____

Thrombocythemia: Overproduction of platelets

Sx: Headache, nausea, vomiting, dizziness, thrombosis

PE:

Dx:

_____   Tx:

_____

_____

Hemochromatosis: **Autosomal recessive**

Complications: Cirrhosis, liver cancer, diabetes mellitus, CHF, arthritis

Sx:

PE:

Dx: Labs:

    Liver biopsy:

_____   Tx:

_____

_____

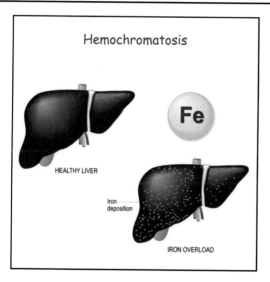

Hemochromatosis

HEALTHY LIVER

Fe

Iron deposition

IRON OVERLOAD

Hemostatis:

Definition:

Explanation:

Medications

_____: MOA = _____

Indication(s)=_____

Side Effects = _____

Types/ Examples = _____

_____

_____

_____: MOA = _____

Indication(s)=_____

Side Effects = _____

Types/ Examples = _____

_____

_____

_____: MOA = _____

Indication(s)=_____

Side Effects = _____

Types/ Examples = _____

_____

_____

_____: MOA = _____

Indication(s)=_____

Side Effects = _____

Types/ Examples = _____

_____

_____

_____: MOA = _____

Indication(s)=_____

Side Effects = _____

Types/ Examples = _____

_____

Medications

_____: MOA = _____

Indication(s)=_____

Side Effects = _____

Types/ Examples = _____

_____

_____

_____: MOA = _____

Indication(s)=_____

Side Effects = _____

Types/ Examples = _____

_____

_____

_____: MOA = _____

Indication(s)=_____

Side Effects = _____

Types/ Examples = _____

_____

_____

_____: MOA = _____

Indication(s)=_____

Side Effects = _____

Types/ Examples = _____

_____

_____

_____: MOA = _____

Indication(s)=_____

Side Effects = _____

Types/ Examples = _____

_____

_____

Renal, GU, Electrolytes

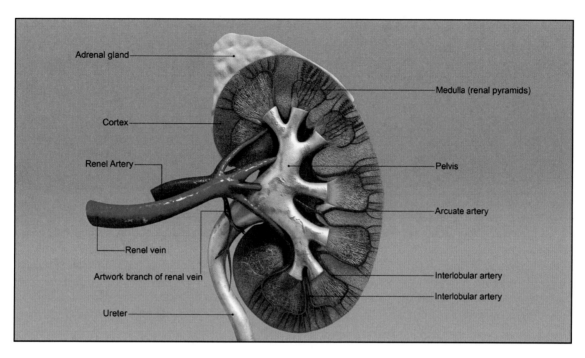

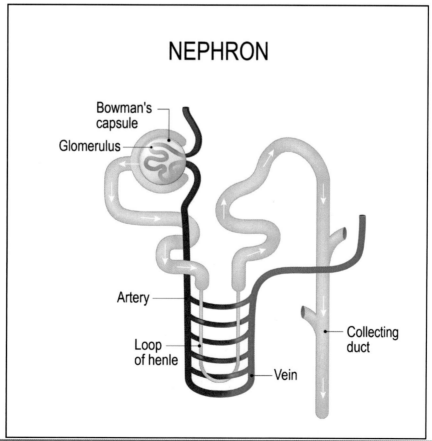

FORMATION OF URINE

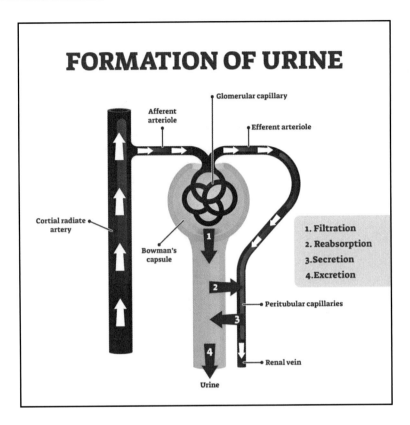

1. **Filtration**
2. **Reabsorption**
3. **Secretion**
4. **Excretion**

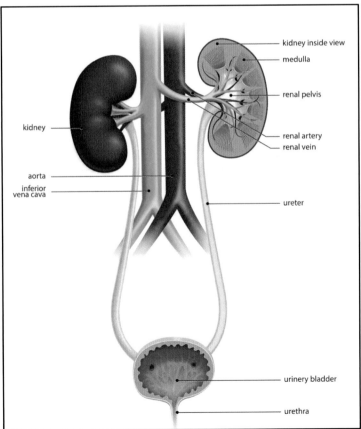

Acute Kidney Injury

Pre-Renal: Decreased perfusion (hypovolemia), renal artery stenosis

Sx:

PE:

Dx: BUN:Cr > 20:1, high osmolality, low FENa

_____   Tx:

_____

_____

Post-Renal: Obstruction, BPH, tumor, stone

Sx:

PE:

Dx:

_____   Tx:

_____

_____

Intra-Renal: Damage to kidney parenchyma

Sx:

PE:

Dx: BUN:Cr < 15:1, low osmolality, high FENa

_____   Tx:

_____

_____

Acute Tubular Necrosis: **Ischemia, drugs, rhabdomyolysis**

Sx:

PE:

Dx: Muddy brown casts

_____   **Tx:**

_____

_____

Acute Interstitial Nephritis: **Infection (strep), drugs (NSAIDs), autoimmune (SLE)**

Sx: Arthralgia, fever, rash, WBC casts, eosinophilia

PE:

Dx:

_____   **Tx:**

_____

_____

Nephrotic Syndrome

Proteinuria > 3.5 g/24-hr, edema, hypoalbuminemia, hyperlipidemia, oval fat bodies

Minimal Change Disease: Idiopathic - usually seen in kids

Sx:

PE:

Dx: Children = clinical, adults = biopsy

_____   Tx:

_____

_____

Membranous Nephropathy:

Sx:

PE:

Dx: Biopsy

_____   Tx:

_____

_____

Focal Segmental Glomerulosclerosis: Most common in black patients

Sx: Primary (idiopathic)
    Secondary (HIV, heroin, obesity)

PE:

Dx:

_____   Tx:

_____

_____

Nephritic Syndrome
Glomerulus inflammation - hematuria, oliguria, hypertension from sodium retention
Damage to the basement membrane

Acute Glomerulonephritis:

Sx: Hematuria, proteinuria, decreased GFR, increased blood pressure, edema

PE:

Dx:

_____   Tx:

_____

_____

Post-Strep Glomerulonephritis: Post strep infection

Sx: Periorbital edema

PE:

Dx:

_____   Tx:

_____

_____

IgA Nephropathy (Berger): **Most common in East Asian patients**

Sx:

PE:

Dx:

_____   Tx:

_____

_____

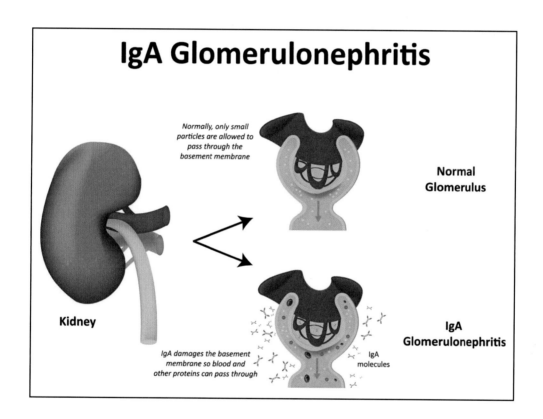

IgA Glomerulonephritis

Normally, only small particles are allowed to pass through the basement membrane

Normal Glomerulus

Kidney

IgA damages the basement membrane so blood and other proteins can pass through

IgA molecules

IgA Glomerulonephritis

Membranous Glomerulonephritis (MGN): **Mostly idiopathic**

Sx:

PE:

Dx:

_____   **Tx:**

_____

_____

Goodpasture Syndrome:

Sx: Hemoptysis

PE:

Dx: Biopsy linear deposits (anti-GBM)

_____   **Tx:**

_____

_____

Chronic Kidney Disease: Low GFR > 3 months

Causes: Diabetes, hypertension

Sx: MAD HUNGER

PE:

Dx:

_____

_____

_____

Tx:

| M |
| A |
| D |
| H |
| U |
| N |
| G |
| E |
| R |

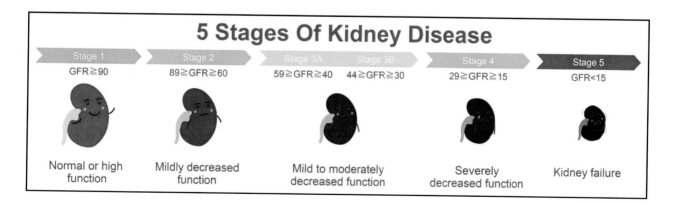

5 Stages Of Kidney Disease

Stage 1	Stage 2	Stage 3A	Stage 3B	Stage 4	Stage 5
GFR≧90	89≧GFR≧60	59≧GFR≧40	44≧GFR≧30	29≧GFR≧15	GFR<15
Normal or high function	Mildly decreased function	Mild to moderately decreased function		Severely decreased function	Kidney failure

Acid Base Disorders

Metabolic Acidosis: **Anion gap = Na- (CL + HC03) < 11**

Anion gap - Sx:

PE:

Dx:

Non-Anion gap - Sx:

PE:

Dx:

_____   Tx:

_____

_____

| M |
| U |
| D |
| P |
| I |
| L |
| E |
| S |

Metabolic Alkalosis:

Causes: Vomiting, diuretics, Cushing's

Sx:

PE:

Dx:

_____   Tx:

_____

_____

Respiratory Acidosis:

Causes: Hypoventilation, COPD, opiates

Sx:

PE:

Dx:

_____   **Tx:**

_____

_____

Respiratory Alkalosis:

Causes: Hyperventilation, pregnancy, anxiety

Sx:

PE:

Dx:

_____   **Tx:**

_____

_____

Electrolyte Imbalance

Hyponatremia: < 135 mEq/L

Sx: Acute = headache, N/V

    Chronic = ataxia

PE:

Dx:

_____

_____   Tx:

_____

Hypernatremia: > 145 mEq/L
Causes: Dehydration, diabetes insipidus

Sx:

PE:

Dx:

_____   Tx:

_____

_____

Hypokalemia: < 3.5 mmol/L
Causes: Diuretics, hyperaldosteronism

Sx:

PE: EKG = flat T waves, U waves, Torsades

Dx:

_____

_____

_____

Tx:

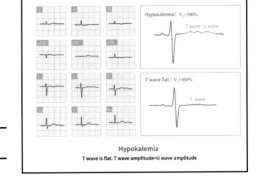

Hypokalemia
T wave is flat. T wave amplitude=U wave amplitude

Hyperkalemia: > 5 mmol/L
Causes: DKA, renal failure, ACE/ARB

Sx:

PE: EKG = peaked T waves, sine wave

Dx:

_____   Tx:

_____

_____

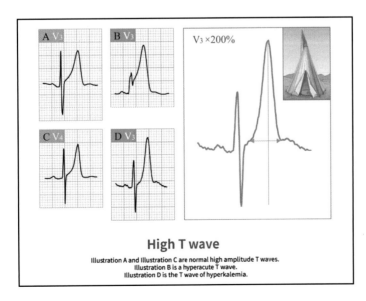

High T wave
Illustration A and Illustration C are normal high amplitude T waves.
Illustration B is a hyperacute T wave.
Illustration D is the T wave of hyperkalemia.

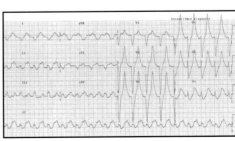

Hypocalcemia: < 8.5 mg/dL total
Causes: CKD, hypoparathyroidism, pancreatitis

Sx:

PE: EKG = long QT

Dx:

_____   Tx:

_____

_____

Hypercalcemia: > 10.5 mg/dL total
Causes: Hyperparathyroidism, malignancy, thiazides

Sx:

PE: EKG = short QT

Dx:

_____   Tx:

_____

_____

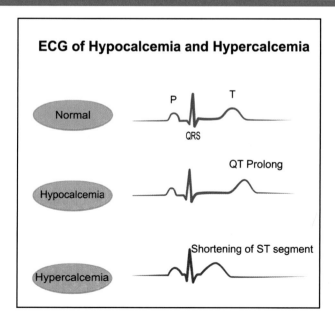

ECG of Hypocalcemia and Hypercalcemia

Normal — P, QRS, T

Hypocalcemia — QT Prolong

Hypercalcemia — Shortening of ST segment

Hypomagnesemia: < 1.8 mg/dL

Causes: Diuretics, alcohol, PPI

Sx:

PE: Long QT, torsades

Dx:

_____   Tx:

_____

_____

Hypermagnesemia:

Cause: CKD

Sx:

PE: EKG = peaked T waves

Dx:

_____   Tx:

_____

_____

Hypovolemia

Isovolumia

Hypervolemia

Renal & GU Infections

Cystitis: Bladder infection (most common cause is E. coli)

Sx:

PE:

Dx: UA

_____

_____

_____

Tx:

Cystitis

Epididymitis: Chlamydia/gonorrhea < 35 years old, E. coli > 35 years old

Sx:

PE: + Cremasteric reflex, + Prehn's

Dx:

_____

_____

_____

Tx:

Epididymitis

Orchitis: Most common cause is mumps

Sx:

PE:

Dx:

_____

_____

_____

Tx:

Inflammation of the testes

Healthy   Orchitis

Prostatitis: Chlamydia/gonorrhea < 35 years old, E. coli > 35 years old

Sx:

PE:

Dx: Digital rectal exam

_____   Tx:

_____

_____

Prostate

Pyelonephritis: UTI that ascends ureters to kidneys

Sx:

PE: Flank pain and/or CVA tenderness

Dx:

_____

_____

_____

Tx:

PYELONEPHRITIS

Urethritis: Most common STI

Sx: Dysuria, discharge

PE:

Dx:

_____   Tx:

_____

_____

Other Kidney Disorders

Nephrolithiasis: **Most common calcium oxalate**

Sx:

PE:

Dx: CT (without contrast)

US if pregnant

Tx:

_____

_____

_____

Hydronephrosis: **Dilation of renal pelvis**

Sx:

PE:

Dx: US then CT

Tx:

_____

_____

_____

Polycystic Kidney Disease: **Autosomal dominant**

Sx: Many people are asymptomatic, HTN, hematuria

PE:

Dx:

Tx:

_____

_____

_____

Renal Arterial Stenosis: **Narrow renal artery**

Sx:

PE: Bruit

Dx: Renal arteriography

_____

_____

_____

Tx:

Renovascular Disease

Vesicoureteral Reflux: **Increased risk for UTI & pyelonephritis**

Sx:

PE:

Dx: Renal US, voiding cystourethrogram (VCUG)

_____   Tx:

_____

_____

Horseshoe Kidney: **Most common renal fusion anomaly**

Sx:

PE:

Dx: US (usually antenatal)

_____   Tx:

_____

_____

Kidney & GU Carcinomas

Wilms' Tumor: Nephroblastoma in children

Sx: Abdominal mass/swelling

PE:

Dx:

_____   Tx:

_____

_____

Bladder Cancer: Most common cause = smoking

Sx:

PE:

Dx: Cystoscopy

_____   Tx:

_____

_____

Prostate Cancer: Most common adenocarcinoma

Sx:

PE:

Dx: Biopsy, MRI, high PSA

_____   Tx:

_____

_____

Screening:

Renal Cell Carcinoma:

Sx: Flank pain, hematuria, mass

PE:

Dx:

_____

_____

_____

Tx:

Testicular Cancer:

Risk Factor: Cryptorchidism

Sx:

PE:

Dx: US, monitor with alpha-fetoprotein

_____

_____

_____

Tx:

Penile Cancer:

Sx: Painless lump or ulcer, lymphadenopathy

PE:

Dx: Biopsy

_____

_____

_____

Tx:

Incontinence Disorders

Stress Incontinence: Coughing, laughing, jumping

Sx:

Dx:

_____   Tx:

_____

Urge Incontinence: Overactive detrusor muscle

Sx:

Dx:

_____   Tx:

_____

Overflow Incontinence: Neurological condition, blockage, or elderly

Sx:

Dx:

_____   Tx:

_____

Mixed Incontinence: Stress + Urge

Sx:

Dx:

_____   Tx:

_____

Functional Incontinence: Physical or mental disabilities

Sx:

Dx:

_____   Tx:

_____

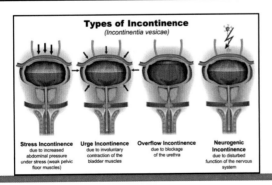

Male Genitalia Concerns

Hydrocele:

Sx:

PE:

Dx: Scrotal US

_____   Tx:

_____

_____

HYDROCELE

NORMAL   HYDROCELE

Epididymis

Testide

Hydrocele

Spermatocele: Epididymal cyst filled with sperm

Sx:

PE:

Dx:

_____   Tx:

_____

_____

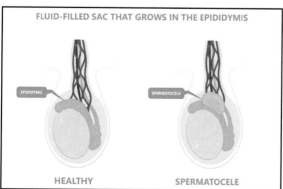

FLUID-FILLED SAC THAT GROWS IN THE EPIDIDYMIS

EPIDIDYMIS

SPERMATOCELE

HEALTHY   SPERMATOCELE

Varicocele: **Dilation of pampiniform plexus**

Sx:

PE: "Bag of worms"

Dx:

_____

_____

_____

Tx:

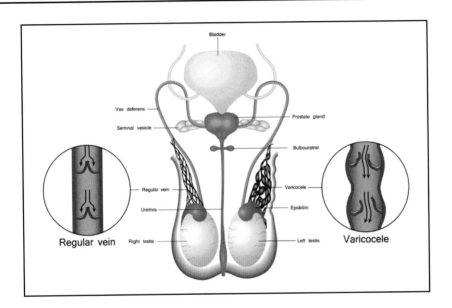

Testicular Torsion: **Acute twisting of spermatic cord EMERGENCY!**

Sx:

PE: Cremasteric reflex absent, bell clapper deformity (predisposition)

Dx:

_____

_____   Tx:

_____

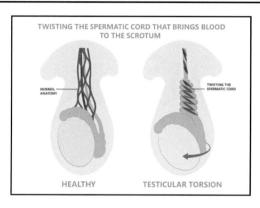

Cryptorchidism: **Undescended testicles**

Sx:

PE:

Dx:

_____

_____   Tx:

_____

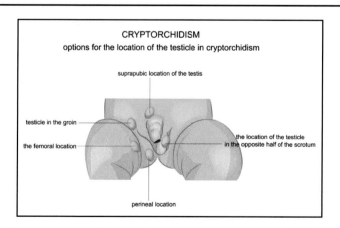

Phimosis: **Can't retract foreskin over glans penis**

Sx:

PE:

Dx:

_____

_____

_____

Tx:

Paraphimosis: **Can't return foreskin EMERGENCY!**

Sx:

PE:

Dx:

_____   Tx:

_____

_____

Priapism:

Sx: Erection for > 2-4 hours without sexual excitement

PE:

Dx:

_____   Tx:

_____

_____

Erectile Dysfunction:

Sx: Difficulty obtaining and/or maintaining an erection

PE:

Dx:

_____   **Tx:**

_____

_____

Peyronie's Disease: Fibrosis of the tunica albuginea

Sx:

PE:

Dx: History & physical

_____   **Tx:**

_____

_____

Epispadias:

Sx:

PE:

Dx:

_____   Tx:

_____

_____

Hypospadias: **Urethral opening on posterior penis**

Sx:

PE:

Dx:

_____   Tx:

_____

_____

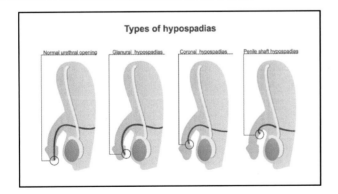

Benign Prostatic Hyperplasia (BPH):

Sx:

PE:

Dx:

_____   **Tx:**

_____

_____

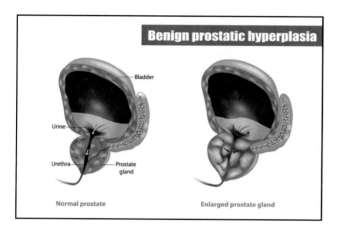

Diuretics: In Cardio

Medications

_____: MOA = _____

Indication(s)=_____

Side Effects = _____

Types/ Examples = _____

_____

_____

_____: MOA = _____

Indication(s)=_____

Side Effects = _____

Types/ Examples = _____

_____

_____

_____: MOA = _____

Indication(s)=_____

Side Effects = _____

Types/ Examples = _____

_____

_____

_____: MOA = _____

Indication(s)=_____

Side Effects = _____

Types/ Examples = _____

_____

_____

_____: MOA = _____

Indication(s)=_____

Side Effects = _____

Types/ Examples = _____

_____

Medications

_____: MOA = _____

Indication(s)=_____

Side Effects = _____

Types/ Examples = _____

_____

_____

_____: MOA = _____

Indication(s)=_____

Side Effects = _____

Types/ Examples = _____

_____

_____

_____: MOA = _____

Indication(s)=_____

Side Effects = _____

Types/ Examples = _____

_____

_____

_____: MOA = _____

Indication(s)=_____

Side Effects = _____

Types/ Examples = _____

_____

_____

_____: MOA = _____

Indication(s)=_____

Side Effects = _____

Types/ Examples = _____

_____

Pediatrics
Milestones

2 months
Closure of posterior fontanelle

_____

_____

4 months
Colic resolves

_____

_____

6 months
Eyes should move in parallel without deviation and be consistently well-aligned

_____

_____

9 months

_____

_____

12 months

_____

_____

15 months
Walks alone

_____

_____

18 months

_____

_____

2 years
Puts 3 words together, feeds oneself, builds a tower with 7 cubes

_____

_____

3 years
Hearing deficit screening (pure tone audiometry)
Annual blood pressures should start at age 3

_____

_____

Reflexes

Moro (Startle)

_____

_____

_____

_____

Asymmetric Tonic Neck Reflex

_____

_____

_____

_____

Palmar Grasp

_____

_____

_____

_____

Rooting

_____

_____

_____

_____

Parachute

_____

_____

_____

_____

Immunization Schedule

Reasons to Delay Immunizations:

_____

_____

_____

_____

Pediatric Cardiology

Newborn Hypertrophic Cardiomyopathy:

Most common cause: Mutations in the genes for sarcomere proteins

Sx:

PE:

Dx:

_____   Tx:

_____

_____

Pediatric Pulmonology

Respiratory Distress Syndrome: Type 2 pneumocytes fail to secrete surfactant

Sx: Tachycardia, nasal flaring, retractions, cyanosis

PE:

Dx:

_____   **Tx:**

_____

_____

Pediatric Gastrointestinal

Meckel's Diverticulum: Most common congenital GI tract anomaly

Sx:

PE: "Currant jelly" stool

Dx: Meckel radionuclide scan or technetium scan

_____

_____   Tx:

_____

Rule of 2's

    2 years old

    2 ft from ileocecal valve

    2" long

    2% of population

Constipation:

Sx: Frequency of stooling depends on age

PE:

Dx:

_____   Tx:

_____

_____

Duodenal Atresia:

Sx:

PE: Bilious vomiting or mild form with distended abdomen

Dx: X-ray with "double bubble"

_____   Tx:

_____

_____

Hirschsprung Disease: **Absence of ganglion cells in colon**

Sx: Failure to thrive, chronic constipation

PE: Abdominal distention

Dx:

_____

_____

_____

Tx:

Hirschsprung's disease

Neonatal Jaundice:

Sx: Yellowing of skin and conjunctiva

PE:

Dx:

_____   Tx:

_____

_____

Pediatric Musculoskeletal

Osteogenesis Imperfecta:

Sx:

PE: Mild form - blue sclera, history of recurrent fractures, presenile deafness

Dx:

_____   Tx:

_____

_____

Osteogenesis Imperfecta — Healthy Bone, Brittle Bone

Duchenne Muscular Dystrophy: Genetic defect on the short arm of the X chromosome. Usually males, diagnosed when toddlers

Sx:

PE:

Dx: CK, genetic analysis

_____   Tx:

_____

_____

Osgood-Schlatter Disease: Tibial Tuberosity Avulsion

Sx:

PE:

Dx: Clinical, X-ray

_____   Tx:

_____

_____

Developmental Dysplasia/Hip Dysplasia:

Sx:

PE: < 3 months + Ortolani/Barlow maneuvers, > 3months + Galeazzi and Klisic test

Dx:

_____   **Tx:**

_____

_____

Torticollis: Twisted neck, usually observed by 2-4 weeks of age

Sx: Head tilted to one side with chin pointed to other side

PE:

Dx:

_____   **Tx: Physical therapy**

_____

_____

Slipped Capital Femoral Epiphysis:

Sx: Hip pain, external rotation/shortening of leg, limp

PE:

Dx: X-ray

_____   **Tx:**

_____

_____

Marfan Syndrome:

Sx: Skeletal abnormalities (tall, joint laxity, pectus deformity), heart/skin/eye abnormalities

PE: + Thumb & wrist sign

Dx:

_____   Tx:

_____

_____

Ehlers-Danlos Syndrome:

Sx: Joint hypermobility, skin hyperextensibility

PE:

Dx:

_____   Tx:

_____

_____

Nursemaid's Elbow: Radial head subluxation

Sx:

PE: Holds affected arm close to body with elbow fully extended or slightly flexed and forearm pronated

Dx: History (pull injury), clinical, X-ray

_____   Tx:

_____

_____

Pediatric EENT

Retinoblastoma:

Sx:

PE: Leukoria (abnormal red-light reflex)

Dx:

_____   **Tx:**

_____

_____

Ophthalmia Neonatorum: Eye infection within first 30 days of life

Sx: Purulent conjunctivitis, swelling & exudate of eyelids

PE:

Dx:

_____   **Tx:**

_____

_____

Pediatric Dermatology

Nevus Simplex (Macular Stain): "Stork Bite"

Sx: Pink/red patches usually on eyelids, glabella, or neck

PE:

Dx:

_____

_____

_____

Tx:

Congenital Dermal Melanocytosis: "Mongolian Spots"

Sx: Blue/grey patches with unclear borders, usually in sacral and gluteal areas

PE:

Dx:

_____

_____

_____

Tx:

Nevus Flammeus: "Port Wine Stains" (capillary malformations)

Sx: Pink/red, flat, blanchable lesions that respect midline, often on face

PE:

Dx:

_____

_____

_____

Tx:

Café-au-lait Macules: **Multiple lesions. Can be a sign of a systemic disorder**

Sx: Flat pigmented lesions, usually a few shades darker than skin

PE:

Dx:

_____   Tx:

_____

_____

Pediatric Endocrinology

Congenital Hypothyroidism:

Sx: Gradual, 3–6-month of age, poor appetite

PE: Enlarged abdomen & umbilical hernia, enlarged tongue, not meeting milestones

Dx:

_____   Tx:

_____

_____

Chromosomal Abnormalities

Klinefelter Syndrome: Extra X chromosome

Sx:

PE: Gynecomastia, tall, thin, wide arm span, small phallus, & small, soft testis

Dx:

_____   **Tx:**

_____

_____

Noonan Syndrome:

Sx:

PE: Short stature, webbed neck, pectus excavatum

Dx:

_____   **Tx:**

_____

_____

21-Hydroxylase Deficiency: Congenital adrenal hyperplasia

Sx:

PE:

Dx: Early morning 17-hydroxyprogesterone level

_____   **Tx:**

_____

_____

Fragile-X Syndrome:

Sx:

PE: Long face, protruding ears, male sex (usually), macroorchidism, macrocephaly, large jaw, frontal bossing

Dx:

_____   Tx:

_____

_____

Down Syndrome: Trisomy 21

Sx:

PE:

Dx: Usually made through prenatal screening, usually clinical after birth, karyotype

_____   Tx:

_____

_____

Prader-Willi Syndrome:

Sx: Large appetite, obesity, decreased cognition, hypogonadism

PE:

Dx: Genetic testing

_____   Tx:

_____

_____

Pediatric Neurology

Niemann-Pick Disease: **2-6 months with progressive neurodegeneration, hypotonia, feeding difficulties**

Sx:

PE: "Cherry red spot" on macula

Dx:

_____

_____   Tx:

_____

Tay-Sachs Disease:

Sx:

PE: Hyperreflexia

Dx:

_____   Tx:

_____

_____

Rett Syndrome: Neurodegenerative disorder of unknown cause

Sx: Almost exclusively in females

PE:

Dx: DNA analysis of MECP2, FOX61, CDKL5

_____   Tx:

_____

_____

Neurocysticercosis: **Tapeworm infection**

Sx:

PE:

Dx: CT and MRI

_____   **Tx:**

_____

_____

Kernicterus: **Brain damage from high bilirubin, develops within 1 year of birth**

Sx: Cerebral palsy, sensorineural hearing loss, gaze abnormality, dental enamel hypoplasia

PE:

Dx:

_____   **Tx:**

_____

_____

Reye Syndrome:

Sx: Lethargy, drowsiness, vomiting

PE: Hyperreflexia, Babinski sign, may have hepatomegaly

Dx:

_____   Tx:

_____

_____

Spina Bifida:

Sx:

PE:

Dx: CT or MRI is definitive test

    Alpha-fetoprotein measured at 16-18 weeks in pregnancy

_____

_____

_____

Tx:

Infantile Spasms:

Sx: Mixed flexor/extensor spasms, sudden flexion of neck, trunk, arms

PE:

Dx: Electroencephalogram (EEG)

_____   **Tx:**

_____

_____

Neuroblastoma:

Sx:

PE:

Dx: CBC, CMP, urine, or serum catecholamine metabolite levels

    Refer to pediatric oncology/surgery for biopsy

_____   **Tx:**

_____

_____

The PA Bible

Pediatric Hematology

Iron Poisoning:

Sx: Initial = vomiting and bloody diarrhea
    Causes localized necrosis & hemorrhage

PE:

Dx:

_____   **Tx:**

_____

_____

Fanconi Anemia: Autosomal recessive

Sx: Short stature, limb abnormalities

PE:

Dx: Labs = macrocytic, pancytopenia

_____   **Tx:**

_____

_____

Increased risk for AML

Homocystinuria: **Disorder of amino acid metabolism**

Sx: Developmental delay, osteoporosis, thromboembolism, marfanoid appearance

PE:

Dx:

_____   Tx:

_____

_____

Cephalohematoma: **Collection of blood between the skull & periosteum - does not cross suture lines**

Sx: Swelling of scalp that doesn't cross suture lines

PE:

Dx:

_____   Tx:

_____

_____

Maternal Substance Use in Utero (Neonatal Abstinence Syndrome)

Cocaine Withdrawal:

Sx: Irritable, tremulous & inconsolable

PE: Increased pulse, small for gestational age, microcephaly, seizures

Dx:

_____   **Tx:**

_____

_____

Alcohol: **Fetal Alcohol Syndrome**

Sx: Thin vermillion border, smooth philtrum, growth retardation, cognitive impairment, hyperactivity

PE:

Dx:

_____   **Tx:**

_____

_____

Barbiturates:

Sx:

PE: Dysmorphic features (short nose & low nasal bridge), limb abnormalities

Dx:

_____   **Tx:**

_____

_____

Opiate:

Sx: Placenta abruption, preterm labor, fetal growth restrictions, tremors

PE:

Dx:

_____   **Tx:**

_____

_____

Heroin:

Sx: Irritable, not feeding or sleeping well, vomiting, loose stools, diaphoretic & high-pitched cry

PE: Fetal growth restrictions

Dx:

_____   **Tx:**

_____

_____

Legg-Calve-Perthes Disease: In MSK

Kawasaki Syndrome: In MSK

Medications

_____: MOA = _____

Indication(s)=_____

Side Effects = _____

Types/ Examples = _____

_____

_____

_____: MOA = _____

Indication(s)=_____

Side Effects = _____

Types/ Examples = _____

_____

_____

_____: MOA = _____

Indication(s)=_____

Side Effects = _____

Types/ Examples = _____

_____

_____

_____: MOA = _____

Indication(s)=_____

Side Effects = _____

Types/ Examples = _____

_____

_____

_____: MOA = _____

Indication(s)=_____

Side Effects = _____

Types/ Examples = _____

_____

_____

Medications

_____: MOA = _____

Indication(s)=_____

Side Effects = _____

Types/ Examples = _____

_____

_____

_____: MOA = _____

Indication(s)=_____

Side Effects = _____

Types/ Examples = _____

_____

_____

_____: MOA = _____

Indication(s)=_____

Side Effects = _____

Types/ Examples = _____

_____

_____

_____: MOA = _____

Indication(s)=_____

Side Effects = _____

Types/ Examples = _____

_____

_____

_____: MOA = _____

Indication(s)=_____

Side Effects = _____

Types/ Examples = _____

_____

Appendix

Bibliography

Images:

iStock. "Royalty-Free Stock Images, Photos and Pictures." iStock, 2021, https://www.istockphoto.com/.

Shutterstock. "Royalty-Free Stock Images, Photos, Vectors, Video, and Music." Shutterstock, 2021, https://www.shutterstock.com/.

Resources:

Epocrates. "Point of Care Medical Applications." Epocrates, 2021, https://www.epocrates.com/.

Wolters Kluwer. "Solutions for Professionals." Wolters Kluwer, 2021, https://www.wolterskluwer.com/.

Williams, Dwayne A,. *PANCE Prep Pearls V3.* Independently published (November 28, 2019)

National Commission on Certification of Physician Assistants. "PANCE Blueprint." NCCPA, 2021, https://www.nccpa.net/become-certified/pance-blueprint/.

The Diagnostic and Statistical Manual of Mental Disorders version 5

Made in the USA
Middletown, DE
02 March 2025

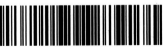

72042525R30331